Epidemic Invasions

**Epidemic Invasions: Yellow Fever and the Limits of
Cuban Independence, 1878–1930**

Mariola Espinosa

The University of Chicago Press :: Chicago and London

Mariola Espinosa is assistant professor in the Section of the History of Medicine at Yale University.

Frontispiece: Map of the Gulf of Mexico. Courtesy of K. J. Carr, 2008.

The University of Chicago Press, Chicago 60637
The University of Chicago Press, Ltd., London
© 2009 by The University of Chicago
All rights reserved. Published 2009
Printed in the United States of America
18 17 16 15 14 13 12 11 10 09   1 2 3 4 5

ISBN-13: 978-0-226-21811-3 (cloth)
ISBN-13: 978-0-226-21812-0 (paper)
ISBN-10: 0-226-21811-2 (cloth)
ISBN-10: 0-226-21812-0 (paper)

Library of Congress Cataloging-in-Publication Data
Espinosa, Mariola.
Epidemic invasions : yellow fever and the limits of Cuban independence,
1878–1930 / Mariola Espinosa.
p. cm.
Includes bibliographical references and index.
ISBN-13: 978-0-226-21811-3 (cloth: alk. paper)
ISBN-13: 978-0-226-21812-0 (pbk.: alk. paper)
ISBN-10: 0-226-21811-2 (cloth: alk. paper)
ISBN-10: 0-226-21812-0 (pbk.: alk. paper)
1. Yellow fever—Cuba—History. 2. Yellow fever—Southern States—
History. 3. Public health—United States—History. 4. Public health—
Cuba—History. 5. Medical policy—United States—History. 6. Medical
policy—Cuba—History. 7. United States—Relations—Cuba—History.
8. Cuba—Relations—United States—History. I. Title.
RA644.Y4E86 2009
614.5'41097291—dc22   2009006776

Contents

Acknowledgments

Early support for this project came from the Institute of Latin American Studies, the Graduate School, and the Department of History at the University of North Carolina at Chapel Hill, which provided a Mowry Research Grant, a Latané Interdisciplinary Summer Research Grant, a Mowry-Waddell Research Fellowship, and a Doris G. Quinn Fellowship. Significant revisions to the manuscript completed during the summer of 2007 were supported by the Jack D. Pressman–Burroughs Wellcome Fund Career Development Award of the American Association for the History of Medicine.

I thank the staff of the Archivo Nacional de Cuba, the Biblioteca Nacional José Martí, the U.S. National Archives, and the Library of Congress. I am especially grateful to María Herminia Pandolfi at the Museo de Historia de las Ciencias en Cuba "Carlos J. Finlay." I also appreciate the help of the Nettie Lee Benson Latin American Collection at the University of Texas at Austin, Davis Library and the Health Sciences Library at the University of North Carolina at Chapel Hill, the Scott Memorial Library at Thomas Jefferson University, Fondren Library at Rice University, the Connecticut State Library, the Houston Public Library, the Claude Moore Health Sciences Library at the University of Virginia, Morris Library at Southern Illinois University, and Jason Bourque,

Alanna Oster, and Alec Heiple at Common Grounds Coffee House in Carbondale.

I have been fortunate to have many friends and colleagues who have read, critiqued, and re-read some or all of this volume, including Steve Bloom, Mike Brown, Kathryn Burns, John Chasteen, Marcos Cueto, Judy Farquhar, Phil Habel, Laura Hatcher, Jim Hevia, Scott McClurg, Celeste Montoya, Lou Pérez, Jr., Leah Potter, Lars Schoultz, and Paul Sutter. Kay Carr graciously volunteered to make the beautiful map. Jean Eckenfels did a superb job copyediting the manuscript. Various portions of this research were presented at the annual meetings of the American Historical Association, the American Association for the History of Medicine, the Latin American Studies Association, and the Southern Historical Association. Parts were also presented at the University of Wisconsin at Madison, Oxford University, the National Library of Medicine, the University of Sydney, and Washington University in St. Louis. I am grateful to the participants of all of these conferences for their helpful comments. I am also thankful for the encouragement and editorial support of Karen Merikangas Darling and the staff at the University of Chicago Press.

Some of the research presented here has been published previously. An earlier version of much of chapter 2 appeared as "The Threat from Havana: Southern Public Health, Yellow Fever, and U.S. Intervention in the Cuban Struggle for Independence, 1878–1898," *Journal of Southern History* 72 (2006): 541–68. Parts of the introduction appeared in a similar form in "A Fever for Empire: U.S. Disease Eradication in Cuba as Colonial Public Health," in *Colonial Crucible: Empire in the Making of the Modern U.S. State,* edited by Alfred W. McCoy and Francisco Scarano (Madison: University of Wisconsin Press, 2009).

I thank Carlos J. Finlay, William C. Gorgas, Jesse Lazear, and Henry R. Carter for their dedication to their work, over a century ago. Finally, I am immensely grateful for the support provided through many years by my family, especially Fred Solt, Katie McCloskey, and Aco Espinosa.

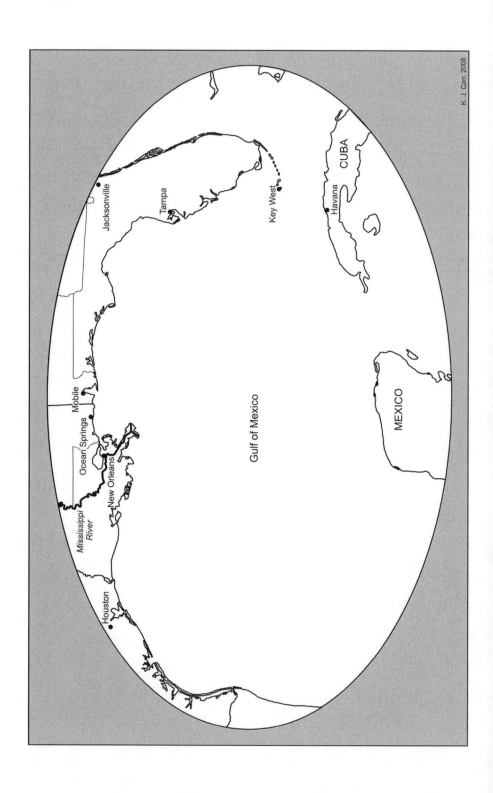

1

Disease and Empire

During Cuba's Ten Years War of 1868 to 1878, the heat and rains of the summer months brought the threat of yellow fever to the battlefront. The "invincible Generals June, July, and August" in this way served as allies for the Cuban Liberation Army in the conflict.[1] Although almost all of the Cuban insurgents were immune to yellow fever due to childhood infection, the newly arriving Spanish troops had never before been exposed to the disease and stood little chance against it. Using yellow fever to their advantage, the Cubans could simply withdraw deep into the countryside during the hot months and leave the Spanish army to its fate.

That fate was indeed horrific. The first sign of the disease was a high fever that lasted for three or four days. During that time, the stricken Spanish soldier suffered from a continuous headache and severe body aches, muscle and joint pain. Suffering from chills and unusually low blood pressure, he was also overcome with nausea. In most cases the fever would then subside, and the patient slowly recovered. In acute cases, however, this relief was like the eye of a hurricane, a deceptive calm. The most fearsome aspect of the disease was imminent. The fever returned, and the body simply began to fail. The soldier was by then screaming and doubled over with pain; the doctors and nurses of the military hospital could only stand by helplessly. The disease attacked internal organs, and, as the liver failed, his skin and eyes turned yellow. He bled from the eyes, nose, mouth, and stomach. He vomited repeatedly, the liquid black with coagulated blood. This last terrifying symptom gave the disease its common name, *vómito negro,* the black vomit. For the afflicted soldier, far from his home and family, there was nothing left to do but wait for death to come.

At the time, it was not known that yellow fever was a virus or that it was transmitted from one victim to the next by mosquitoes. The principal carrier of the disease, a frail, house-inhabiting species known first as *Culex* and then as *Stegomyia* in the nineteenth century, and as *Aedes aegypti* today, prefers to lay its eggs in small, artificial containers of clear water, thereby concentrating yellow fever epidemics in urban settings where these conditions were present; other species perpetuate the disease among monkeys in the rainforests of the Amazon and parts of tropical Africa.

Anyone who had seen the way yellow fever ravaged its victims or even heard secondhand accounts of its effects was likely to conclude that his best chance lay in staying as far away from it as possible. But the Spanish soldiers had little choice other than to go where they were ordered, and as they sailed to the battleground in Cuba, they knew that most of them would never make the trip back. In the city of Havana alone, 11,590 people, the vast majority of them Spanish troops, died of yellow fever during the Ten Years War.[2]

When yellow fever first reached Cuba is unclear, but it had been endemic in Havana since before the British occupied the city in 1762 and had come to the Caribbean aboard slave ships from Africa at least a century before that.[3] The disease was always present in the city: records show that during the nineteenth century very few months passed without the disease taking at least a handful of lives. During a typical summer month, yellow fever could claim one hundred victims. And when unrest on the island brought large numbers of Spanish soldiers to the city, men who had never before been exposed to the disease, the death rate from yellow fever could increase by fivefold or more.

Despite its decimation of the Spanish army, yellow fever turned out not to be so advantageous for the cause of Cuban independence after all. By the end of the Ten Years War, although scientific knowledge of the disease was limited, it was evident that yellow fever could spread from place to place and travel aboard ships, boats, and trains. This meant that the disease was a threat to the health of those port cities engaged in trade with Havana and so also to the cities and towns of the interior that were linked to these ports. The southern United States, just across the Gulf of Mexico from Cuba, frequently suffered yellow fever epidemics during the second half of the nineteenth century, and nearly all of these epidemics had been traced back to the island. Many other diseases routinely caused greater mortality, but because yellow fever killed in such a horrific fashion and could take thousands of lives in just a few short weeks, word of an outbreak often triggered mass panic.[4] Many barricaded their towns against all outside contact to avoid contagion; others fled to the countryside until winter frosts brought the epidemic to an end. Even a relatively small epidemic could halt business activity across much of the region from midsummer through the fall.[5] Faced with repeated invasions of epidemic yellow fever from Havana in its southern states, the U.S. government confronted Cubans with the prospect of an epidemic of invasions of their island by U.S. troops.

Of course, other factors also shaped U.S. policy toward Cuba in the late nineteenth century. Many U.S. citizens were motivated by a genuine humanitarian desire to liberate Cubans from the chains of Spanish tyranny.[6] Within government circles, the extensive and growing economic ties between the United States and Cuba and a long-standing fascination with the idea of annexing the island were important influences.[7] The substantial U.S. interest in eradicating yellow fever in Cuba, however, has been overlooked. This book demonstrates that the devastating power of the yellow fever virus had a crucial and long-lasting impact on the relationship between the two nations.

Disease and Public Health in History

The history of disease, medicine, and public health in Latin America has attracted increased attention from historians of the region in recent years.[8] A few of these works have described how, as in politics, economics, culture, and many other matters, the United States has exerted a profound influence on the public health policies of Latin American countries.[9] But this historiography has thus far developed in isolation from the broader literature on how disease and efforts to control it in colonial contexts are distinctly different from those where foreign domination is absent. Bringing insights from the study of colonial public health in other parts of the world to modern Latin America is among the goals of this book.

Historians of public health in many noncolonial contexts have shown that epidemics frequently serve to illuminate divisions within a society, particularly along lines of class and race. The biological characteristics of most epidemic diseases ensure that they will affect different groups of people to varying degrees; this differential impact, in turn, leads to a range of opinions regarding causes and appropriate responses to outbreaks. In Europe, for example, both the cholera that swept over the continent five times during the nineteenth century and the authorities' measures against the disease exacerbated social tensions and dramatically revealed stark divisions between rich and poor and between town and countryside.[10] Similarly, turn-of-the-century efforts to eradicate smallpox in Brazil through obligatory vaccination touched off riots that reflected long-standing grievances of the urban middle and lower classes against the country's agricultural and commercial elite.[11] In the U.S. South, yellow fever epidemics revealed tensions between classes and races. New Orleans was regularly afflicted by them, but nearly all of the city's affluent native-born citizens were immune to the disease as a result of childhood infection. Instead, it was the newly arrived Irish working class that suffered the highest mortality from yellow fever, leading the elite to blame poor whites for the insalubrious reputation of their city. This view, coupled with reports that blacks contracted only mild cases of the disease, provided many wealthy New Orleanians with a further justification for their continued reliance on black labor in the southern climate.[12] As these examples and countless others show, epidemics and efforts to cope with them "betray deeply rooted and continuing social imbalances."[13]

Colonialism, however, changes the nature of the social imbalances exposed by epidemic diseases. Rather than bringing antagonisms based on class or race within a nation to the foreground, epidemics and the public health measures they provoke tend instead to underscore the power inequalities between colonizer and colonized. In India, for example, where the cholera epidemics that aggravated class conflicts across Europe originated, the spread of the disease from Bengal to the rest of the subcontinent did not inflame animosities between rich and poor.[14] Rather, as the East India Company had only recently consolidated its control in the region, the occasionally violent responses to cholera epidemics and British efforts to control the disease reflected "the wide social, religious and political gulf" that divided Indian subjects and their new British rulers.[15] Similarly, the smallpox and cholera epidemics that swept through coastal Algeria soon after the French invasion in 1830 caused little tension among the groups that made up indigenous Algerian society but only "reinforced the didactic relationship between occupier and occupied."[16] Whether bubonic plague in French Senegal, sleeping sickness in the Belgian Congo, or malaria in British West Africa, the principal fault lines revealed by epidemic disease in colonial societies were those between conqueror and conquered.[17]

Like much of the Caribbean basin, Cuba came to be politically and economically dominated by the United States in the late nineteenth and early twentieth centuries. Repeated U.S. military occupations and political interventions coupled with massive U.S. investment made the island effectively a colony of the United States.[18] In this setting, yellow fever in Havana and the public health policies pursued by the U.S. government in Cuba to control the disease necessarily highlight not those differences that divided Cubans but instead those between Cuba, on the one hand, and the United States, on the other. It is these national differences that make up the focus of this book.

Motivating Colonial Public Health

Scholars of colonial public health have long recognized that efforts by foreign powers to control epidemic diseases primarily served the interests of the colonizers rather than the colonized. These interests were both economic and political. For the economy of the empire, disease posed two threats. First, epidemic diseases menace the commercial intercourse that makes the domination of foreign lands profitable. Colonial public health measures therefore frequently had as their goal the protection of trade. The famed Liverpool School of Tropical Medicine, for example, was founded at the end of the nineteenth century by the city's commercial community to prepare medical officers for the British colonies. The shipping magnate Alfred Lewis Jones, who served as the first chairman of the board, made the school's purpose clear at its inception: it was "an investment, and we expect dividends from it."[19] Second, epidemics could debilitate the native workforce upon which the colonial economy depended. Where labor was in chronically short supply, as in central Africa, protecting the health of miners, farm workers, rubber tappers, and the host of other laborers demanded by the colonial economy became a matter of importance to the authorities.[20]

There were also two political concerns that motivated colonial health efforts. The first consideration was protecting troops and administrators from disease, which was paramount to the maintenance of colonial rule. The use of quinine to combat malaria among colonial troops, for example, is frequently credited with allowing the European colonization of Africa to succeed.[21] The consequences to the colonial enterprise of failing to protect soldiers' health were clear: the massive French expedition to put down the Haitian Revolution in 1802 failed because 25,000 of its 35,000 men succumbed to yellow fever in nine months, and an earlier effort by the British to seize the colony was abandoned after losing three-fifths of its soldiers to disease.[22]

The second political concern was that colonial public health provided a legitimating justification for the domination of foreign lands and peoples both to the publics of colonizing powers and to the colonized. Efforts to combat epidemic diseases provided colonizing powers with evidence to assure skeptical observers among their own citizens and in the international community that the colonial enterprise was fundamentally benevolent. Public health was an integral part of the "civilizing mission" that served as the rationalization for most imperialist ventures; moreover, advances in health were both readily observed and difficult for critics to deny. That the process of colonization—by inducing population movements into zones of infection, changing the environment in ways favorable to the proliferation of disease, and creating new routes for the spread of pathogens—was itself the cause of many epidemics was almost always overlooked by contemporary proponents and detractors of imperialism alike. The need to burnish a public image badly tarnished by revelations of the mistreatment of the Congolese was a principal motivation for the decision of King Leopold II to mount an investigation into sleeping sickness in the Belgian Congo; decades later, Belgian colonial administrators continued to point to their successes in controlling the disease as a justification for empire.[23]

Public health efforts also sought to convince subjugated peoples of their own inferiority and, therefore, the desirability of continued colonial rule. As they carved out a sphere of influence in southwest China in the 1890s, the French established medical dispensaries to check the spread of bubonic plague and win the confidence of the local populace. The resulting improvements in public health convinced many of the superiority of Western ways and "proved to be an effective way to gain the sympathy of both the elite and the common people" for French domination of the region.[24] Of course, colonizing powers did not always achieve their goal of gaining support among their subjects for continued colonial rule through public health measures. Frantz Fanon famously described how the French failed in their attempts to do so in Algeria. "The fact is," he wrote, "that the colonization, having been built on military conquest and the police system, sought a justification for its existence and the legitimization of its persistence in its works." But the colonized Algerians, perceiving that "the French medical service in Algeria could not be separated from French colonialism in Algeria," rejected the French doctors along with the rest of the colonial administration.[25]

The relative importance of these four motivations to a particular colonial effort to combat a disease depends on specific characteristics of the malady concerned: most directly, its method of infection, which determines both its propensity to spread and the identity of its most frequent victims. Contagious diseases and diseases whose vectors are well suited to travel most often triggered imperial responses aimed primarily at protecting trade. The policies adopted by both British and French colonial authorities against cholera and bubonic plague in the latter decades of the nineteenth century were expressly directed at preserving commercial intercourse, while the health of the local labor force and that of the imperial presence was of only secondary concern.[26] On the other hand, diseases whose pathologies confined them to particular environments—such as sleeping sickness and malaria—instead prompted measures directed mainly at safeguarding local workers and the colonial authorities. Dangers to trade in such cases could be ignored without risk to the imperial project. Whatever the balance among these motivations in fighting a particular disease, it was the interests of the empire, not those of colonial subjects, that impelled disease control efforts.

Yellow Fever, Cuba, and U.S. Domination

Attention to the history of public health, this book reveals, provides important insights into the U.S. domination of Cuba. The next chapter describes how endemic yellow fever in Havana and its periodic spread to the U.S. South had become a source of apprehension to the U.S. government long before the United States declared war on Spain in 1898. When the passengers of a steamship that traveled from Havana to New Orleans in 1878 were allowed to disembark without passing through quarantine, the yellow fever they carried touched off the worst epidemic in U.S. history. That summer, yellow fever ravaged the population of New Orleans and worked its way up the Mississippi Valley as far north as St. Louis. Over twenty thousand people died from the disease, and the panic that ensued caused economic losses across the region of up to two hundred million dollars. In an attempt to ensure that yellow fever would not threaten the United States again, U.S. sanitarians began to study its causes and developed a system of quarantine along the gulf coast to prevent its entry. Both efforts failed. Bacteriology was then the cutting edge of medical science, but it could provide little insight into the cause of yellow fever, a viral disease. Quarantine restrictions were costly, difficult to implement, and subject to lapses when state and local authorities put the benefits of trade above the risk to public health. As U.S. commercial relations with Cuba expanded, unease in the United States about the threat of yellow fever grew as well; this anxiety was heightened further by the rapid increase in the disease on the island after the Cuban War of Independence began in 1895. When the deteriorating conditions in Havana produced an epidemic that again paralyzed the economy of the southern United States in 1897, U.S. politicians and diplomats joined public health officials in considering yellow fever to be a source of tension with Spain, a tension that contributed to the U.S. declaration of war in 1898.

The U.S. intervention in Cuba in 1898 put the United States in a position to take action on yellow fever in Havana after decades of concern. When the U.S. Military Government was established in December 1898, it moved quickly to clean the island in an effort to rid it of the disease. In chapter 3, I discuss the sweeping efforts made by the occupation government to eradicate yellow fever at its source. As it was believed that yellow fever lived in filth and in materials infected by people sick with the disease, wide-ranging exertions were directed at cleaning the streets, buildings, and harbor of Havana. Because it was known to be an urban disease, U.S. troops were stationed outside of the island's cities. Additional camps were built outside of Havana for immigrants and other nonimmune people in an effort to minimize the exposure of the population capable of contracting and spreading the disease. Although these measures improved the overall health of Havana's residents, yellow fever continued to strike in even the most affluent and cleanest of the city's neighborhoods.

The failure of the initial sanitary measures led to renewed efforts to understand and control yellow fever on the island. Chapter 4 explores the attempts undertaken by the U.S. occupation government to determine the cause of yellow fever in Havana. Combining the theory of a Cuban doctor, Carlos J. Finlay, who argued that a single species of mosquito was the only means by which yellow fever was transmitted from one victim to the next, with the findings of a U.S. sanitarian, Henry R. Carter, who established that ten to twelve days elapsed between an initial infection of a previously disease-free location and subsequent secondary cases, the U.S. Yellow Fever Commission designed a series of experiments that convincingly established that mosquitoes alone conveyed the disease. This breakthrough led to a revolution in the methods used by the sanitary authorities in Havana. Although the measures that kept the city clean were maintained, the U.S. occupation government's health and sanitation policies came to focus on the destruction of mosquitoes and their breeding places. By the end of 1901, there was no yellow fever in Cuba.

The maintenance of sanitation measures to prevent yellow fever was a critical concern when the United States ceded control of the island to the Cubans in 1902. Chapter 5 examines the ways in which issues of disease and sanitation affected U.S.-Cuban relations after the first U.S. occupation of the island. It begins by recounting the heated debates in both Cuba and the United States that preceded the inclusion of a sanitation clause to the Platt Amendment to the Cuban Constitution of 1902, which demanded that Cubans maintain the public health measures instituted by the U.S. occupation government and raised the threat of U.S. intervention if Cuban sanitary conditions declined. Sanitation remained a major source of tension between the two countries during the first five years of Cuban independence, particularly after yellow fever reappeared on the island. By the time political unrest led to a second U.S. occupation of Cuba in 1906, yellow fever was again epidemic. The new U.S. Provisional Government responded by expanding the sanitation measures that had been imposed in Havana during the first occupation to the entire breadth of the island. By the end of the U.S. intervention in 1909, Cuban government officials and sanitarians had learned that keeping the island free of yellow fever was critical to maintaining the independence of their new nation from the United States.

Cubans, however, did not accept this arrangement without complaint. In chapter 6, I illuminate the ways in which Cubans voiced their discontent with the burden imposed on them by the United States for the public health of the region. Since the end of the second intervention in 1909, Cubans faced constant accusations in U.S. publications that they cared little about sanitation, were generally dirty, and purposefully hid cases of yellow fever in Cuba. Rather than passively accepting these purported justifications for close U.S. supervision of the island, health officials in Cuba zealously denied them. They instead pointed to the existing deficiencies in the U.S. public health apparatus, which failed to even attempt the steps necessary to make a yellow fever outbreak in the U.S. South impossible. Cubans also contested the U.S. claims of all credit for the scientific achievements that led to the eradication of yellow fever from the island. They insisted on due acknowledgment of the fact that the work done by their compatriot Carlos J. Finlay was fundamental to the success of the effort. Cubans knew themselves to be in no way inferior to the United States in terms of public health, and they therefore refused to accept that the U.S. imposition of sole responsibility for regional sanitation on their country was legitimate.

The book concludes by demonstrating that the inherently colonial nature of U.S. efforts against yellow fever in Cuba is paradigmatic of subsequent U.S.-sponsored public health measures in Latin America. As in Cuba, these later measures were prompted by the spread of U.S. economic interests. Teams of U.S. Army sanitarians fought the disease in Panama to allow the construction of the canal to the Pacific Ocean and in the key port of Veracruz during the Mexican Revolution. The Rockefeller Foundation, at the urging of the U.S. military, undertook the work of eradicating yellow fever from the Americas after 1914. The informal empire of the United States in Latin America, no less than overt European colonialism in Africa and Asia, depended on public health to safeguard the colonizer's interests in trade, protect its troops and labor force, and justify its domination of foreign lands. And U.S. colonial public health began with the fight against yellow fever in Havana.

2

The Pre-Occupation with Cuba

Cuba, as its prosperity and commerce increased, has become the greatest nursery and campaign ground of one of man's most ruthless destroyers. Itself most sorely afflicted, it annually disseminates to other lands, as from a central hell, disease and death. . . . Had the nation human enemies possessing like characteristics, no knowledge of their country or of their conduct would be deemed too minute or superfluous; and, in this light, the present report on yellow fever has been written.   **Stanford E. Chaillé, "Report to the United States National Board of Health on Yellow Fever in Havana and Cuba"**

: : :

In September and October of 1897, the southern United States was gripped by a terror that shuttered businesses, paralyzed trade, and caused tens of thousands of people to abandon their homes and flee for their lives: yellow fever had returned. Decades of experience had taught southern health officials the source of this dreaded disease. The 1897 yellow fever epidemic, like many outbreaks before it, was of Cuban origin. Unlike previous episodes of infection, by the end of 1897 the U.S. government was determined to end the ongoing threat to the health and economy of the southern states posed by yellow fever in Cuba. The island would be invaded and the disease stamped out at its source.

After weeks of suspicion, the news broke on September 7, 1897: there was yellow fever in New Orleans.[1] U.S.

Army soldiers stationed there were quickly ordered to abandon the city and evacuate to the safety of Fort McPherson in Atlanta.[2] Within a week, "King Jack" had brought virtually all movement on the railroads to a halt for three hundred miles around; only a few passenger trains were rolling, each carrying a full load of terrified refugees bound directly for the safety of northern points.[3] The steamship trade similarly came to a halt. The U.S. Mint in New Orleans was shut down because there was no way to ship out the coins and currency.[4] Many attempted to argue that only recent arrivals to the city were panicked, but there was soon no denying that even native residents were scared. When the Board of Health began to convert a school to an emergency yellow fever hospital for "that class of unfortunate citizenship, who, being stricken with the yellow fever, may not find themselves in a position to be taken care of at home," fearful inhabitants of the surrounding neighborhood set fire to the building and repeatedly cut the hoses of the firefighters who were attempting to save the structure.[5] By the end of the epidemic two months later, 1,675 cases of yellow fever had been diagnosed in the city, and the disease had claimed more than two hundred lives.[6]

Yellow fever—and so panic—spread across the South. When several suspicious cases of fever occurred in the town of Edwards on September 13, the citizens of nearby Jackson, Mississippi, evacuated en masse. The next day, half of the residences of the state capital stood empty, and when seven cases at Edwards were definitively identified as yellow fever the following morning, most of the remaining inhabitants joined the exodus.[7] The state government, both daily newspapers, and all of the city's businesses, except for the grocery store, were closed for the duration of the epidemic. The remaining residents adopted an absolute quarantine: armed guards were stationed at all approaches to prevent anyone, even returning residents, from entering the city, regardless of whether they held a doctor's certificate attesting to their good health.[8] As further insurance against infection, a railroad bridge along the line between the city and Edwards was set on fire and completely destroyed.[9] The quarantine at Jackson was successful—no cases of yellow fever developed in the city—but until it was lifted six weeks later, the city was completely idled.

When word of the yellow fever outbreak in New Orleans reached Texas, the state government quickly imposed quarantine against all infected points.[10] Initially, the port at Galveston actually benefited from steamship traffic rerouted from New Orleans. On September 23, however, a fatal case of yellow fever was identified at Beaumont, to the northeast of Houston near the Louisiana border.[11] The news caused an eruption of local quarantines. When a suspicious case was found in Houston a few days later, hundreds of refugees swarmed the city's train stations.[12] Even yellow fever experts dispatched to Texas from New Orleans by the U.S. Marine Hospital Service (USMHS) were turned back in western Louisiana by a Winchester-toting mob that "threatened to tear up the track and burn the bridges before they would allow the train to go through"; the doctors eventually reached Houston from the north via St. Louis.[13] When the disease reached Galveston, quarantine against the city forced the steamship companies to close entirely until the end of the epidemic.[14] Only fifteen cases of yellow fever were diagnosed in Texas, with only a single death, but commerce was disrupted for weeks on end.

The city leaders of Atlanta took a different stance with regard to the epidemic. Confident that the city's climate would prevent yellow fever from gaining a foothold, they announced that those fleeing from infected locations would be welcomed. During the first weeks of the epidemic, several hundred refugees took up this invitation each day, brought from across the South by the few trains still running. The arriving refugees were checked for symptoms before being permitted to enter the city, and any suspicious cases were removed to a quarantine camp outside the city for observation and treatment.[15] Fortunately, the judgment of Atlanta's city leaders proved sound; the city remained free of yellow fever.

Other southern cities found the risk of contagion posed by the refugees in Atlanta to be too great to hazard. In Alabama, the cities of Huntsville, Decatur, Selma, Montgomery, and Mobile promptly raised a rigid quarantine barring all arrivals from Atlanta. Chattanooga, Charleston, and Wilmington quickly followed suit, as did many towns in Georgia. All backed up their proclamations, reminding at gunpoint those who forgot the prohibition of travel from Atlanta.[16] Business, as a result, slowed to a crawl. "The dead line has been drawn," complained the *Atlanta Constitution* after weeks of quarantine, "the mails have been practically stopped, the railways have all but suspended operations, and all forms of interstate traffic have been as good as abolished."[17] The effects of the yellow fever epidemic dragged down the stock prices of southern companies, and the entire New York market followed.[18]

In Alabama, however, the quarantine would prove as ineffective as it was costly. By mid-October, yellow fever reached the capital and panic ensued as thousands fled the city. "When old Vesuvius erupted and the people flew from the fast-creeping yellow lava, the terror in Pompei was probably little more intense than it has been here since yellow fever has been announced to exist in Montgomery," reported one observer, "The stampede is positively astonishing."[19] Alabama cities and towns that had earlier quarantined against points in neighboring states then turned against each other; the railroads and most other businesses soon came to a halt statewide.[20]

The epicenter of this human and economic catastrophe was the re- sort town of Ocean Springs in Mississippi. Vacationers returning home to New Orleans and Mobile brought the disease with them; efforts by doctors and health officials in those cities to conceal the outbreak in order to prevent panic only succeeded in allowing the disease to spread. The sickness had earlier run through the inhabitants of Ocean Springs, slowly marching up one street and then the next during July and August; the town's Catholic and Presbyterian churches also appear to have been foci of infection. Most of the earliest cases were among children. Several children contracted well-marked cases of yellow fever by mid-June; on June 2, the son of one Mrs. Gonzales was the first to be diagnosed. Mrs. Gonzales was Cuban, and her home also served as the gulf-coast head- quarters for Cuban insurgents who smuggled people and contraband between the United States and Havana, surreptitiously avoiding both the nearby Ship Island quarantine station and the Spanish authorities. In so doing, they also brought with them yellow fever, which was always and notoriously present in Havana.[21]

The threat posed to the southern United States by yellow fever in Havana had first attracted government attention a generation before 1897, in the wake of the 1878 Mississippi Valley epidemic. Unlike the 1897 outbreak, which had spread beyond Ocean Springs just two months before hard frosts brought it to an end, the 1878 epidemic had raged the entire summer. From New Orleans the disease spread up the river and outward along railroad lines, ultimately claiming victims in more than one hundred cities and towns. Over one hundred twenty thousand people were stricken; more than twenty thousand perished. The economic damages were also disastrous. Commerce ground to a halt as panicked townspeople imposed self-help "shotgun" quarantines. Total economic losses were estimated to be at least one hundred million dollars; many put the figure as high as twice that amount.[22] U.S. health officials were convinced that the origin of the infection was Havana, noting that with the end of the Ten Years War on the island that year, hundreds of refugees had fled to New Orleans from Cuba. Many con- temporary sanitarians identified the precise source of the epidemic as the ship *Emily B. Souder,* a steamer from Havana that had been allowed to discharge its passengers in New Orleans before passing through quarantine; two of these travelers were among the first to be diagnosed with yellow fever.[23]

Yellow fever had to be understood and controlled in order for the U.S. South to prosper. The epidemic prompted intense research on the disease. In the summer of 1879, the newly formed U.S. National Board of Health sent a group of experts, the Havana Yellow Fever Commission, to Cuba. Headed by New Orleans physician Stanford E. Chaillé, the group was charged with studying yellow fever in Havana and other localities on the island where the disease was believed to be prevalent: "It is believed," Chaillé wrote, "that if mankind is ever to be protected from this scourge this must be accomplished by stamping it out at its very source."[24] The commission's chief purpose was to determine both the sanitary conditions that allowed yellow fever to flourish in Cuban ports and the measures, if any, that might be instituted to prevent ships bound for the United States from being infected with the disease. With the assistance of Cuban physicians, it also studied the symptoms associated with yellow fever.[25]

It was widely believed at the time that yellow fever was a disease that lived in and was transmitted by filth, so the commission focused on the sanitary conditions of Cuba. It found sanitation in Havana and in other Cuban cities to be practically nonexistent. Most housing was poorly constructed, with little ventilation, and very crowded: many families lived in one-room apartments in ramshackle tenement houses. Less than one-third of Havana's population lived on paved streets. Most houses had simple privies for the disposal of human waste. "The effluvia therefrom pervades the houses, and the fluid contents saturate the soil and the soft porous coral rocks on which the city is built. Hence, all well-water is ruined, and every ditch dug in the streets exhales an offensive odor. Thus Havana may be said to be built over a privy."[26] What sewers existed emptied into the harbor and, with little circulation between the harbor and the open sea, the waste simply settled to the bottom of the bay.

The mission of the Yellow Fever Commission was not only to study yellow fever but also to suggest policies that would protect the United States from the importation of the disease from Cuba. The simplest remedy to the problem of the spread of yellow fever from Havana to ports in the U.S. South was to encourage Spain to sanitize the city and make it safe for commercial vessels. But there was little chance that Spain would prove willing—or even capable—of taking up the issue. The sanitary infrastructure thought necessary, including a clean water supply, a sewer system, paved streets, and a thorough dredging of the harbor, was estimated to cost at least $20 million, and the Spanish government, despite brutally high levels of taxation, was already unable to pay even the interest on its debts.[27] As Spain would not take the steps required to control yellow fever in Havana, the task would fall to the Cubans themselves, the commission deduced: "Until the accomplishment (which the present generation will not live to witness) Havana will continue to be a source of constant danger to every vessel within its harbor, and to every southern port to which these vessels may sail during the warm season."[28] In the meantime, the United States had little choice but to protect itself from Cuba.

For this purpose the commission recommended several measures, beginning with a strict quarantine system. The Spanish government had itself established a "severe" quarantine in order to prevent yellow fever infection from traveling from Cuba to Spain. Lasting from May 1 to October 1 each year, it affected all ships coming to Spain from Cuban ports, even those with bills of health.[29] As the Spanish quarantine seemed to be successful, the commission suggested that a similar quarantine was a viable option for the United States as well.[30] Commerce could suffer, since restricting trade in this manner could reduce the amount of products sold and bought between the United States and Cuba. But the commission concluded that trade that did not occur during the yellow fever season would simply be conducted during the rest of the year.

Ships that had been in Cuban ports, the commission suggested, should be disinfected and their cargoes quarantined before being allowed to enter U.S. ports. Moreover, because ships docked at Havana's wharves were more likely to become infected than those that remained farther out in the harbor, the U.S. doctors recommended that ships anchor away from the shore.

Although the National Board of Health dissolved when the U.S. Congress failed to reauthorize it in 1882, its quarantine recommendations were gradually adopted. A patchwork of local, state, and federal quarantine provisions grew and was integrated by the end of the 1880s. Quarantine stations operated by the USMHS off the coast of Mississippi and Georgia and at Key West, together with state facilities in New Orleans, Mobile, and along the Florida coast, disinfected incoming ships and provided a defensive line against the importation of yellow fever.[31] But yellow fever seemed to ignore the system of controls established after 1878. Sanitarians worried that business interests would always find a way to avoid costly public health measures that infringed on their profits. Despite the dangers, commercial interests too frequently sought to avoid costly delays in quarantine by putting pressure on local officials.[32] In 1888, despite the network of disinfection stations, an epi-

demic in Jacksonville again spread panic throughout the U.S. South. As
had happened a decade earlier, local quarantines disrupted commerce
and had a devastating impact on business.[33] The origin of the infection was again traced back to Havana. The American Public Health
Association, composed of public health officials from Canada, Mexico,
and the United States, urged the U.S. government to take action in face
of this recurring threat from Havana. So, President Grover Cleveland
dispatched George Sternberg, a U.S. Army bacteriologist who had been
part of the 1879 commission, to Cuba to investigate the biological cause
of the disease. Sternberg concluded that the various bacteria previously
suggested to cause yellow fever had no correlation with the occurrence
of the disease.[34] The cause of yellow fever remained unknown.

   In December 1892, the Committee on Immigration of the U.S. Senate, along with the Senate Committee on Epidemic Diseases, and in
cooperation with the House Committee on Immigration and Naturalization, established a committee "to examine into the conditions of immigration from Cuba and the West India Islands, and the danger of the
importation of epidemic and contagious diseases into the United States
through immigrants from those islands."[35] The assembled senators and
congressmen visited Havana, Key West, and Tampa. They found that
travel between Cuba and Florida was extensive: as many as one hundred thousand people were estimated to travel back and forth each year.
Given the unsanitary conditions in Havana and the constant presence of
yellow fever in the city, this traffic posed a great risk to the United States.
"The sanitary condition of Havana is a perpetual menace to the health
of the people of the United States," the committee declared.[36] Moreover,
the situation was likely to worsen further in the years to come:

> The island of Cuba, lying in the Gulf of Mexico and almost
> touching the shores of the United States, was regarded by all
> the great statesmen of our earlier history as an outpost of the
> United States, the key to the Gulf, and the necessary place of
> guard and protection for its commerce. It is one of the most
> fertile regions in the world, and has a future before it of great
> development. Its commerce with the United States must con-
> tinually increase, and the interests of the American people will
> become more closely connected with the health and prosperity
> of the people of the island.[37]

The importance of Cuba to the commerce of the United States would
only increase further "because of the certainty of the opening of one or

more transits by waterways across the States of Central America," the legislators pointed out.[38] In order to protect the United States from the spread of contagious disease from Cuba, they recommended that Congress grant the president an appropriation of one million dollars and the authority to suspend all immigration and commerce when necessary until any threatened epidemic had passed. Endemic yellow fever in Havana could not be tolerated indefinitely, they concluded:

> The day is near at hand when 100,000,000 people will inhabit the United States, the most prosperous, free, and intelligent people of the world, cultivating peaceful relations with all nations, but powerful enough to demand justice, right, and protection for all the people of the Americas and the adjacent islands, and with the duty incumbent on them to initiate the policies which will best conduce to their just and fair commercial intercourse, to their mutual protection, and their progress in all the arts and sciences which promote the wellbeing of the great body of their people.[39]

The threat posed to the United States by Havana's endemic yellow fever grew rapidly in the years that followed, but not as a result of the expansion of commerce as predicted by the congressional committee.

When Cuba's War of Independence began with the Grito de Baire on February 24, 1895, thousands of Spanish soldiers were sent to the island. The influx of these troops, the vast majority of whom had never before been exposed to yellow fever, led to a sharp increase in cases of the disease. "Nearly one-third of all the soldiers imported from Spain in Cuba have been sick and many of them have died," reported the *New York Times* on April 4. "Havana had sixty-six new cases of yellow fever yesterday. Of these, the majority were Spanish soldiers. All Americans are leaving Cuba, fearing the fever."[40] U.S. sanitary authorities watched the situation closely. "The insurrection in Cuba causes a condition of affairs unpleasant for the health officials to consider. Marine hospital officials declare that the shipment of several thousand new Spanish troops into Cuba, at this season of the year, none acclimated, is bound to precipitate an epidemic of yellow fever, the ill effects of which must, in a degree more or less severe, be felt in this country," the paper reported.[41]

There was good reason for worry. The Cuban insurgents relied on a strategy of controlling the countryside, generally avoiding direct conflict, and counting on yellow fever attacking the Spanish soldiers who controlled the island's cities, but the Spanish apparently did not believe the disease was a cause for concern. One Spanish diplomat went so far as to assert that yellow fever would in fact provide the Spanish army with the tempering it needed to wage war in the tropics: "The 'green' troops will, of course, have the yellow fever. They will need it to become acclimated, so that they can equal the rebel negroes in endurance."[42] By the end of 1895, 7,085 Spanish soldiers would be diagnosed with yellow fever, and 2,796 of them, 40% of the sickened, would die from the disease.[43]

This high mortality rate among the soldiers afflicted with yellow fever and the evident spread of the disease among patients attracted the attention of the Spanish army's doctors to the condition of the military hospitals. The chief of the Sanitary Corps of the Spanish army in Cuba, Major General Cesáreo Fernández de Lozada enacted changes meant to address the issue soon after arriving on the island in November 1895. He closed the filthy San Ambrosio military hospital, which adjoined Havana's notoriously insalubrious harbor, and relocated its patients to a new facility named Alfonso XIII, situated on a breezy hill on the outskirts of the city and isolated from other buildings. Alfonso XIII provided separate wards for yellow fever victims, a measure not employed elsewhere that reduced the chances of spreading infection among other patients and contributed to the lowest mortality rate of Havana's military hospitals for the duration of the war.[44]

The situation was closely watched in the United States. In May, Surgeon General Walter Wyman of the USMHS toured the quarantine stations along the south Atlantic seaboard to ensure that they were prepared for the increased threat of yellow fever from Cuba.[45] He went on to Havana to examine the conditions there firsthand. No matter how dire the situation may have seemed, it was critical to avoid panic. Upon returning to Washington, he sought to assuage fears of an immediate epidemic: "at the present there is no danger of an outbreak of yellow fever in Cuba, despite the presence of a large number of unacclimated Spanish troops," he announced. "The danger will arise later in the season, and it was to prepare against it that his trip was undertaken."[46]

The danger began to increase in June. The USMHS became concerned that a fleet of small fishing boats sailing from Havana was avoiding the quarantine measures that protected the U.S. South. Not only did these boats enter U.S. waters along the Gulf and south Atlantic coasts to fish, the service warned, but they also smuggled tobacco, rum, and other goods. As smugglers, they necessarily came ashore at night, far from legal entry points, and without passing through disinfection at any quarantine station. These fishing boats were reported to dock in a part of the harbor in Havana known for its particularly unsanitary condition, directly above the outlet of the sewer serving the Cabañas barracks. Further, the crews were often new arrivals to Havana: they were not immune to yellow fever and so were susceptible to infection. The health officials feared that both the crews and their illicit merchandise could carry yellow fever infection to the United States. In addition, with the outbreak of war on the island, there was the possibility that Cuban insurgents and others would use the fishing boats to travel to the United States. "The danger of the introduction of yellow fever by this means has always been considered imminent, but this year it is particularly threatening by reason of the insurrection in Cuba," Wyman reported.[47]

To meet this threat, the U.S. Treasury Department dispatched four revenue cutters to patrol the coastal areas. These cutters sought out the illegal fishing boats by patrolling the coast and stopping at points where the Cuban vessels were known to congregate. When encountering any foreign ship, the cutters acted as quarantine regulators. Any foreign vessel found to be lacking the appropriate health documents was "seized and carried to the nearest quarantine station, there to be disinfected and held five days after disinfection, and afterwards to be delivered to the collector of the nearest port of entry."[48] Because the revenue cutters were too large to navigate the inlets where the Cuban fishing boats were likely to hide, they were outfitted with small, motor-driven launches that went out several days at a time to patrol these shallow waters.[49] Each cutter was also assigned a sanitary inspector from the USMHS, effectively making the ships mobile quarantine stations. The revenue cutter patrols were maintained for the duration of the Cuban insurrection.[50]

These precautions seemed to be successful in preventing the importation of yellow fever from Havana into the southern United States during 1895, but as the war in Cuba intensified, Wyman grew even more concerned about the deteriorating health conditions on the island and the increasing threat they presented to the United States. In the conclusion to the USMHS annual report for 1895, he expressed his fears.[51] The port of Havana, he noted, was notoriously unsanitary and was each year the site of numerous cases of yellow fever. Moreover, ships regularly left Havana for dozens of ports in the United States.

The main problem in Havana, Wyman contended, was the harbor itself. The narrow entrance to the harbor prevented the tide from entering, and most of the harbor shore was made up of swamps, marshes, pools, and other shallow areas where the water did not circulate.[52] The wharves where U.S. vessels frequently docked were especially unsanitary. "There the wharves are not only a continuation of the city," D. M. Burgess, the USMHS sanitary inspector stationed in Havana, observed, "but they are in very much worse sanitary condition than it is, for the sewers of the town debouche right under them, the timbers which support them entrapping all manner of filth and rendering what little tide-water current there might be entirely inefficient for any cleaning purpose."[53] The Tallapiedra and San José wharves, which managed much of the trade between the United States and Cuba, were located in what was identified as one of the most dangerous areas in the harbor: immediately above the sewer outlet of the military hospital where Spanish soldiers with yellow fever were treated. The Tallapiedra wharf, Burgess indicated, "in addition to its close proximity to the ever-infected military hospital with its dangerous sewerage, has all the liquid filth from all the slaughter houses of the city passing slowly under and near it. This is the most dangerous wharf here, and is the one to which many American and British vessels go to discharge lumber." Only slightly less dangerous was the San José wharf, "with its hospital at either end and sewer from the military barracks, has also city sewers emptying under it."[54]

The dangers posed by docking at these wharves, USMHS Surgeon General Wyman insisted, could not be overstated. Many ships' captains were known to pay a substantial premium to unload to lighters in the open bay and so avoid the near-certain occurrence of yellow fever brought by tying up at a wharf. The threat was not limited to the sailors themselves but also to the people of the United States, Wyman noted. Ship captains, wary of incurring yet another expense, often refused to leave a sick crewmember behind when sailing from Havana; the city's hospitals charged between two and three hundred dollars to cover all possible expenses of a foreign patient. For this reason, many sailors infected with yellow fever were brought back to U.S. ports, forming "one of the most fruitful sources of danger to our Southern seacoast cities."[55]

Sanitarians and engineers had offered many plans to correct the insalubrious conditions of the harbor in Havana, from dredging and building canals to building walls and filling up the marshy areas. Wyman, however, considered it unlikely that the Spanish administration would undertake such a massive project in a time of insurrection. There was only one way to secure "immunity from this dread pestilence" and still be able to continue commercial trade with Cuba, he concluded: "by intelligent sanitary work in our Southern seaports, namely, the providing of a thorough system of drainage and sewerage, good water supply, and municipal cleanliness," and "also by demanding of our neighbors that their ports shall be made to be of as little danger to the people of the United States as the ports of this nation are to them."[56] After all, he stressed:

> Since 1862, more than a quarter of a century ago, our shores have been infected with yellow fever in each of twenty-six years. The source of the infection is known positively for nineteen years. Of the 19 yearly visitations 16 have been traced definitely to Habana, 2 to Cuba and the West Indies, and 1 to Honduras. The records further show that in some years a number of places have been infected independently of one another from Habana, as, for example, in 1862, Key West, Fla., and Wilmington, N.C.; in 1871, Cedar Keys, Tampa, and New Orleans, and in 1873, New Orleans and Pensacola.[57]

In short, the source of yellow fever infection in the United States was Havana.

As conditions worsened in Cuba, Wyman urged the U.S. State Department to take action to force Spain to correct the unsanitary conditions in Havana that were widely believed to cause the city to be a focus of yellow fever "which annually threatens life and commercial prosperity in a large portion of the United States."[58] The situation was dire. Many U.S. sanitary officers, Wyman indicated, insisted that the only safe course of action was to eliminate all contact with Cuba.[59] The United States should not continue to tolerate this state of affairs, Wyman wrote: "I wish as a sanitary officer, having in view the safety of the United States from visitations of yellow fever, to protest against these conditions, so strikingly in contrast with the sanitary enlightenment of the age, and so threatening to the commerce and lives of the people of other countries, and particularly our own."[60]

Secretary of State Richard Olney relayed Wyman's objections to the Spanish Minister at Washington, Enrique Dupuy de Lôme. The threat of yellow fever from Havana, Olney stressed, called for "sanitary precautions and measures of effective quarantine which bear onerously upon the intercourse of the United States and the chief commercial port of the Island of Cuba, through which the bulk of our Antillean commerce passes." The situation could not be ignored for long, Olney warned: "Sooner or later the problem of attacking the pestilential conditions which exist and have existed for more than a century at Habana will demand the attention not only of Spain, but of other endangered countries, with a view to devising an effective remedy for the state of things disclosed in Surgeon General Wyman's report, and the gravity of the situation invites timely attention and action."[61]

Olney's warnings, however, went unheeded. With the war dragging on, the yellow fever situation only worsened in 1896. The Spanish strategy of concentrating troops in Cuban cities had provided an ideal environment for the spread of yellow fever, and more and more nonimmune Spanish troops were arriving on the island. From 90,000 at the beginning of the year, the Spanish forces numbered 110,000 by April; 130,000 by September; and 200,000 by November. Some thirty thousand Spanish soldiers contracted yellow fever in 1896, completely overwhelming the existing military hospitals and drawing more attention from U.S. observers.[62] Although the government rigorously censored public health statistics, the New York Times reported that "still it is known that the malady has extended all over the island, and the death rate is very great. In some places, as for instance, the military line, it is known that there are hundreds attacked with this terrible disease, and that it is increasing daily in alarming proportions."[63] Press reports of the spread of yellow fever in Cuba continued throughout the summer.[64]

By September, the disease had infected so many Spanish troops in Havana that the authorities converted the sugar storehouses in Regla, across the harbor from the city, into makeshift yellow fever hospitals.[65] This step only heightened the concerns of USMHS officials: they believed the buildings were certainly contaminated and any sugar stored there before export to the United States would become infected, increasing the likelihood that the disease would spread to southern ports.[66] The San Ambrosio hospital, which had been closed during the first year of the war because it was deemed too filthy and contributing to yellow fever, was reopened. The Spanish army also emptied Havana's civilian hospitals for its own use, and even appropriated an orphanage, turned out the children, and crammed it full of beds for the sick troops.[67]

These events prompted Wyman to step up his campaign to force Spain to control Havana's endemic yellow fever. At the September 1896 meeting of the American Public Health Association, he proposed a resolution directed squarely at the Spanish administration in Cuba. At his urging, the association's members resolved, "Whereas yellow fever is believed to be the most subtle and dangerous of all epidemic diseases . . . That it is the duty of every government possessing seaports thus infected to institute such engineering and other sanitary measures as will remove this menace to the seaports of other nations."[68] He reinforced this message in an address at the Pan-American Medical Congress in

Mexico City the following month. After stating his case that Havana was uniquely responsible for spreading yellow fever to ports throughout the western hemisphere, Wyman argued that the nations of North and South America should no longer idly submit to this threat. Havana was not the only port infected with yellow fever, he acknowledged, but addressing the most dangerous port first would yield the greatest gain in safety. "The time has come," he said, "when we should submit no longer to this annual trepidation concerning yellow fever and when the restrictions to commerce caused by infected seaports should be removed. And we should not fail to impress upon others their responsibility with regard to this public sentiment."[69]

The yellow fever situation in Cuba was indeed cause for worry. The war in Cuba provided ideal conditions for the spread of yellow fever in Havana and across the island (see fig. 1). Havana suffered from 300 to 400 yellow fever deaths per year from 1889 to 1894, but the civilian toll reached 553 in 1895, the first year of the war, before jumping to 1,282 in 1896 and 858 in 1897.[70] In the province of Santa Clara, where yellow fever caused approximately 150 deaths annually from 1889 to 1894, the disease claimed 540 lives in 1895, then tripled to 1,552 deaths in 1896 and 1,469 deaths in 1897.[71] In the port city of Santiago de Cuba, deaths from yellow fever rose from less than one hundred per year in 1893 and 1894 to 664 in 1895 and 976 in 1896. Observers in Santiago de Cuba confirmed that the primary cause of the sharp increase in yellow fever mortality was the number of unacclimated Spanish troops brought into the city to combat the insurgency. Between 1895 and 1896, 1,601 Spanish soldiers were killed by yellow fever in Santiago de Cuba, but the disease claimed only 65 civilian lives during those two years, not many more than the average before the war.[72]

Other Cuban cities followed the same pattern of infection. In Cienfuegos, it was reported that while there were 46 deaths of yellow fever in 1894 and 34 in 1895, the disease claimed 301 lives in 1896 and 115 in 1897.[73] As in the years before the war, yellow fever was rare in Matanzas in 1895, when there were only 5 reported deaths from the disease in the city. But with the arrival of large numbers of Spanish troops and civilians relocated from the countryside yellow fever fatalities reached 626 in 1896 and 127 in 1897.[74]

The Spanish authorities could not keep up with the increasing numbers of soldiers coming down with the fever. Lacking the ability even to provide beds for all of the sick soldiers, in 1897 Spanish military doctors responded to pressure to reduce the number of yellow fever deaths among the troops by employing one of the few measures avail-

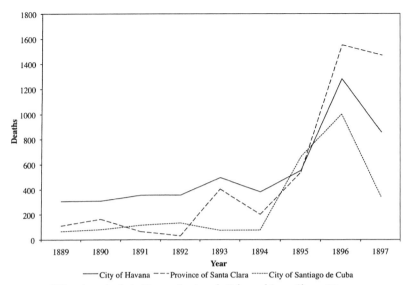

FIGURE 1 Yellow fever deaths in Havana, Santiago de Cuba, and Santa Clara, 1889–97

able to them: they began reporting the deaths as having been caused by other diseases. W. F. Brunner, the inspector of the USMHS stationed in Havana, reported that according to the official Spanish statistics on yellow fever, it appeared "that this disease is decreasing. This appearance is not real. [T]he deaths from yellow fever are being absorbed by those credited to other diseases."[75]

Brunner found that the most common diagnosis used to cover up yellow fever was the so-called "pernicious" fever. Declaring a case to be pernicious fever had been a favorite means of hiding yellow fever, and temporarily delaying the panic it provoked, for doctors across the U.S. South for decades. When yellow fever was present in a southern town, it was common that "all cases of the disease, until it becomes epidemic, are reported as 'pernicious malaria,' 'bilious intermittent,' or some other kind of fever, so that strangers may not be frightened away and in order that the commerce of the locality may not be jeopardized by the establishment of quarantines."[76] After investigating personally, Brunner concluded that Spanish "deaths from pernicious fever should also be counted as yellow fever."[77]

Malaria was also frequently blamed for deaths caused by yellow fever. Ángel de Larra y Cerezo, head of the Alfonso XIII military hospital, pointed out that malaria in Cuba, though extremely widespread and debilitating, was only very rarely fatal and caused just 306 deaths in 1896—a mortality rate of less than 1 percent of the cases severe enough to be hospitalized.[78] Nevertheless, the deaths of approximately 7,000 Spanish troops were attributed to pernicious and malarial fevers in the military hospitals in 1897.[79]

The number of soldiers dying from yellow fever was further obscured by shipping many victims back to Spain: the official records for 1897 did "not include hundreds of deaths that occurred among certain troops sent back to Spain" in the final stages of the illness. "Having observed those departures from Habana," Brunner wrote, "I can safely say that 10 per cent of the 30,000 invalided home were destined to an early and positive death."[80] Judging from the outrage in the Spanish press over the "cemetery ships" arriving from Cuba laden with soldiers dying of yellow fever, it seems that his estimate was indeed conservative.[81]

Despite the increased incidence of yellow fever in Cuba, the USMHS succeeded in preventing yellow fever from spreading to the U.S. South for the first two years of the Cuban struggle for independence. In 1897, however, its measures failed. The revenue cutter patrols notwithstanding, some Cubans frequently evaded the quarantine and landed in the United States along the gulf coast at night. It was one of these groups of insurgents that brought yellow fever to the resort town of Ocean Springs, Mississippi.[82] The result, as reported by Wyman, was a "well-defined epidemic of yellow fever in Ocean Springs, [which] spread to other states, with results which must still be fresh in the minds of all here present, of shotgun quarantines, disturbances of business, interruption of passenger traffic, hardships imposed on travelers, and all the other unhappy concomitants of a yellow fever epidemic."[83]

That Cuba was the origin of the epidemic was widely reported in U.S. newspapers. The disease "was carried over from Havana by certain mysterious Cuban visitors," the *New York Daily Tribune* noted.[84] "Take the yellow fever scare in the south. The contamination was brought by refugees from Cuba," declared the *Atlanta Constitution*. The U.S. government, the paper argued, should "demand of Spain that Cuba be purged of the conditions which have made it a plague spot for years and a menace to surrounding countries."[85]

The overt response of the U.S. government, however, was to send yet another team of U.S. scientists to Cuba to study the cause of yellow fever.[86] The USMHS doctors, Eugene Wasdin and H. D. Geddings, made little progress before increasing tensions between the United States and Spain interrupted their research.[87] Other U.S. policymakers, unwilling to tolerate the continuing economic hardships suffered by the South due to Spanish neglect of the issue of yellow fever, had undertaken a more direct approach to remedying the problem.

Even before Wyman mounted his campaign to bring pressure on Spain to eliminate the threat to the U.S. South posed by yellow fever in Havana, many others had advocated stronger measures. Federal government officials, state sanitarians, and newspaper editors were among those who argued that the United States would not be free from this menace until it seized Cuba and itself eradicated the infection in Havana. These calls to action only grew louder as conditions on the island deteriorated and yellow fever again spread from Havana to the South.

The idea that the United States should acquire Cuba so as to ensure the health of the South had been considered in government circles for many years.[88] In the summer of 1884, Republican presidential candidate James G. Blaine was reported to promise that if elected he would "acquire Cuba by purchase, stamp out the yellow-fever there by methods which our energy and superior skill will provide, and cultivate the commerce of our Southern ports."[89] That same summer it was widely reported that a State Department official had suggested "the real reason why the United States should obtain possession of Cuba is that it may furnish Havana with a system of drainage and stamp out yellow fever."[90]

Soon after the Jacksonville epidemic of 1888, an officer of the Pennsylvania Board of Health again called for the annexation of Cuba in order to control the threat of yellow fever being imported from the island. After describing the constant travel between the United States and Havana, "one of the most notorious breeding-places of yellow fever," and arguing that the only way to control the disease was to establish a good system of sewers and drains in the city, he noted that "there is no hope that the Spanish government will ever undertake a work of this magnitude for a dependency." Under these circumstances, the introduction of yellow fever into the United States would continue to be a frequent occurrence. The U.S. government should act, he concluded: "A single widespread epidemic of yellow-fever would cost the United States more in money, to say nothing of the grief and misery which it would entail, than the purchase-money of Cuba."[91]

But the Spanish government had steadfastly rebuffed the notion of selling Cuba, and when insurrection again erupted on the island in 1895, its efforts to put down the rebellion made clear that it would not relinquish control without a fight. Yellow fever flourished in the devastation that ensued. The *New York Journal,* solidly in favor of U.S. intervention in the conflict, observed the increasing risk these conditions posed to the United States. The paper added pointedly, "The danger might be removed if American civilization with its sanitary ideas were to control the island."[92] With the outbreak of yellow fever in the South in 1897, the *Journal* was more explicit. "At at least one of the points at which yellow fever has appeared on our gulf coast, and probably at the others, the disease is of Cuban origin. It prevails at Havana all the time," it railed: "Spanish shiftlessness and official imbecility have maintained at that port a nuisance that has threatened the health of the world. . . . The extirpation of Spanish rule in Cuba is a sanitary measure essential to the safety of the United States."[93]

Not surprisingly, many in the South shared this view. "It would have been, indeed, remarkable if the warm season of 1897 in our gulf coast States should have passed and yellow fever not have made its appearance," opined the *Houston Daily Post* when the presence of the disease in New Orleans became known:

> The communication with Cuba has been so close, so extensive and in a majority of cases so secret, we should naturally expect an infected visitor to slip in. Indeed, Cuba under Spanish rule, without anything like good sanitation, is a standing menace to the health of the Southern States of the Union and the Washington government has been repeatedly urged to present the Cuban question in this aspect among others to the Spanish authorities. That any heed would be given our protests in the premises is extremely problematical, and it is likely that the great Southern scourge will continue to find a habitat in Cuba and annually require extra quarantine precautions on our part, until American good sense and sanitation have free course in the Ever Faithful Isle.[94]

By the time the epidemic spread to Texas, the paper was even more blunt: "If annexing Cuba will result in eradicating yellow fever and quarantine, by all means let us annex it at once."[95]

The epidemic led even the *Atlanta Constitution* to abandon its previous opposition to U.S. involvement in Cuba. The USMHS planned to fumigate every infected building across the South in an attempt to eradicate the disease and prevent a recurrent epidemic the next yellow fever season. Nevertheless, "it is idle to close our eyes to the fact that, so long as the United States has no authority to fumigate Havana just so long will quarantines and fumigations on our coast and inland cities infected by refugees prove ineffectual." Even if yellow fever were eliminated in the South, the next ship arriving from Havana, where the disease was always present, would only infect it again. The city's natives were immune to the disease; even if the resources necessary to eliminate it were available, they had little reason to take the trouble.

> If there were no other argument in favor of the annexation of Cuba by the United States this would be entirely sufficient. It involves the safety of tens of thousands of men, women and children, to say nothing of the sacrifice of millions and millions of money in the way of trade and commerce. . . . When our government has control of the sanitation of Havana and other Cuban ports, the danger of infection in this country will be reduced to a minimum; but until that time comes it will be impossible to prevent the appearance of the plague on our shores. It is not only a matter of dollars and cents, it is a matter of life and death. So long as the port of Havana blows the infection in this direction (through a funnel as it were), just so long will our measures of precaution, no matter how scientific and thorough, prove entirely ineffectual.

The fumigation effort could perhaps have yielded the desired result for a year or two, allowing the people who fled in panic to return to their homes and prostrated businesses a chance to rebuild. The paper opined, however, that any sense of security gained from the measure would be false. At any time, a ship from Havana arriving in a southern port could reverse all of this progress, costing the lives of thousands and again throwing trade and commerce across the South into complete disarray. There was only one solution, according to the *Constitution*: "It is necessary, therefore, in the interests of all who are affected by an epidemic in the south that Cuba should be annexed, to the end that the plague, which has existed on the island for so many years, should be stamped out."[96]

The federal government had recently, but quietly, reached a similar conclusion: the United States had no choice but to intervene in Cuba to end the threat of yellow fever. Some senators and congressmen had been advocating that the United States end Spanish rule over the island for this reason since the outbreak of fighting. Senator Wilkinson Call of Florida, for example, argued that, "Just as long as [Cuba] is kept under Spanish domination just so long will it be a constant menace to the health of the people of the United States."[97] But by the autumn of 1897, the McKinley administration agreed.

As yellow fever raged in the South, a new U.S. minister to Spain arrived in Madrid. Charged with making the U.S. case for an immediate resolution of the war in Cuba to the European powers before delivering an ultimatum from President McKinley to the Spanish government, Stewart L. Woodford approached the ambassadors of Great Britain, Russia, and Germany.[98] Foremost among the concerns he expressed was the ongoing threat of yellow fever that the continuing hostilities posed to the United States. Woodford reported to Secretary of State John Sherman:

> I pointed out that nearly every epidemic of yellow fever in the United States has originated in Habana or at some point in Cuba, from which the disease has spread to our coast. I told him that owing to the bad sanitary conditions of Cuba and the peculiar formation of the harbor of Habana, which is never thoroughly washed out by the tides, this danger is great even in times of peace. That in war and with the present neglect of sanitary precautions at Habana and throughout Cuba, the danger is increased terribly. I see from the telegrams of the last few days that an immediate confirmation of my statements has come from points in Mississippi and Louisiana and possibly in Georgia and Texas.[99]

Only after emphasizing the constant danger of yellow fever did Woodford mention the personal losses of U.S. citizens who had invested in the island and the horrors of the Spanish concentration camps. Woodford stressed to each of the ambassadors that the role of the U.S. government was to secure peace in Cuba so as to protect the lives and commercial interests of U.S. citizens.[100] Years of fighting in Cuba had already led to one yellow fever epidemic in the southern United States. The U.S. government was poised to take action to prevent another.

On April 25, 1898 the United States declared war on Spain. The *New York Times* reminded its readers that yellow fever in Havana had long provided sufficient justification for the war: "Any country which would carelessly allow such a disease-breeding centre to affect the ships of the world without any effort to improve the conditions deserved nothing better than the most severe and summary punishment."[101] The Spanish forces in Cuba, worn down by years of war with Cuban insurgents and ravaged by disease, quickly collapsed when faced by the fresh U.S. troops. By the end of July, the war in Cuba was effectively over. After two decades of apprehension caused by the threat posed to the southern United States by yellow fever from Havana, the United States at last had an opportunity to root out the disease at its source.

3

Fighting the Yellow Scourge: Initial Sanitation Reforms in Cuba

There was one great object we had in view in taking possession of Cuba, and that was the ridding of it of yellow fever. **Major William C. Gorgas, "Address Delivered before the District of Columbia Medical Association"**

: : :

After decades of growing concerns in the United States for Havana's endemic yellow fever, the war of 1898 had put U.S. authorities in a position to take action. During the first two years of the occupation of Cuba, the military government undertook a wide range of policies to eliminate at its source the disease that had threatened the southern states. These efforts were obsessively focused on sanitation. In order to control yellow fever, the occupation government cleaned streets and buildings, dredged the busiest harbors of the island, quarantined boats and immigrants, disinfected mail and shipments, and isolated nonimmunes from possible sources of infection. Although all of these measures conformed to the most advanced understandings of disease provided by the recent development of bacteriology and germ theory, yellow fever—caused by a virus—posed a challenge. The sanitation of Havana, in the end, would not stop yellow fever.

During the first half of the nineteenth century, the prevailing understanding of yellow fever within the medical community was that the disease, like many others, originated in miasma. That is, breathing a sort of bad air or vapor, something that emanated from a particular location, caused people to fall ill. It was thought that when the weather was sufficiently hot and humid, the filth commonly found in cities of the day—the accumulated human waste, the effluvia of slaughterhouses, the dead animals left to rot in the streets—spontaneously emitted the sickening gas. Disease was therefore an attribute of place; the location itself was sick. Cleaning and sanitizing these specific perceived sources of illness was thus the established method of controlling an outbreak.

Theories of origins of disease began to change in the middle of the century. In the United States, the 1840s and 1850s witnessed a series of yellow fever epidemics in cities that were rarely afflicted, such as Charleston and Norfolk; conditions in these locations at the time of the outbreaks did not appear to be unusual, casting doubt on miasma theory.[1] An additional blow to miasma as an explanation of disease came with John Snow's observations of the 1854 cholera epidemic in London. A physician, Snow noted that cases of the disease could be traced to water sources that were contaminated by the excrement of earlier victims. Cholera was no longer seen as bound to a particular location that exuded miasma, but instead as an illness that could travel through the water supply.[2]

Other scientific advances contributed to moving further away from the miasma theory and toward a germ theory of disease, most notably those of Louis Pasteur in the early 1860s and Robert Koch in the 1870s. Pasteur was able to show that disease did not generate spontaneously and that a microorganism that did not fit through the pores of a filter could generate disease. Koch provided additional observations and developed a set of criteria, or postulates, that must be present in order to conclude that an ailment is caused by a germ. Even though germ theory was not immediately accepted as the explanation for diseases, the techniques recommended for controlling diseases understood as caused by germs were also those that had been used to eliminate sources of miasma: cleaning up and sanitizing. Therefore, in the later nineteenth century, sanitation was at once the most advanced and sophisticated method of controlling disease and also the prescription of those doctors and public health officials who were not yet convinced by the most recent scientific developments.

If there remained any doubt that yellow fever was not a disease bound to a particular place, the 1878 Mississippi Valley epidemic dispelled it. Havana was the source of infection, but the disease had traveled by ship to New Orleans and then spread upriver and out along the railroad lines. The course of the epidemic and the recent development of germ theory led to a new conception of the disease: rather than miasma spontaneously generated in a place, yellow fever was caused by contact with fomites—objects that had been infected with the vomit or excrement of earlier victims.

The advances in medical knowledge, the concern with fomites, and the focus on sanitation that they suggested were quickly shown not to be a promising route to control yellow fever. Working with the 1879 commission that the U.S. National Board of Health sent to investigate the causes of yellow fever in Havana, Carlos J. Finlay, a Cuban physician, made observations that indicated that the disease did not follow the principles of germ theory. Among other contributions, Finlay conducted a study of the workers who maintained Havana's cesspools, expecting them to be the most likely victims of the disease. What he came across was completely the opposite. These workers, he found, suffered a very low rate of yellow fever, casting doubt on the idea that the disease, like cholera, was spread by contaminated human waste. The workers, in constant contact with the filth thought to carry the yellow fever germ, were in fact healthier than the average resident of Havana.[3] Despite this evidence that something else was the cause of yellow fever, few saw a convincing alternative to germ theory, the forefront of scientific knowledge of the day. This meant that when United States forces gained the opportunity to stamp out yellow fever in Havana, their efforts would be driven by an obsession with the sanitation and cleanliness of the city.

This opportunity came in the wake of the war with Spain. The Spanish forces in Cuba, sick and exhausted from three years of fighting the Cuban rebels, had quickly collapsed when confronted with fresh U.S. troops. The surrender of Santiago de Cuba scarcely two weeks after the landing of the U.S. Army effectively ended Spanish resistance on the island. The Treaty of Paris that formally marked the end of the conflict required Spain to relinquish its claim to Cuba but—unlike Puerto Rico, Guam, and the Philippines—not to cede the island to the United States.[4] This provision was in accordance with the joint resolution of the U.S. Congress that authorized the war, which declared that the United States had no intention of exercising any control over Cuba "except for pacification thereof" and that it would then "leave the government and control of the island to its people."[5] As a practical matter, however, the United States would not consider Cuba to be pacified until after yellow fever was under control in Havana and the rest of the island.

Therefore, when the U.S. Military Government of Cuba began operations on January 1, 1899, it was charged, among other things, with ridding the island of yellow fever.[6] Among its first steps was the development of a comprehensive and long-lasting campaign of cleaning and sanitizing Cuban streets. In the larger cities of the island, sanitation was in the hands of the military government's Department of Engineers, while in smaller towns the task fell to the local public works departments of the civil provincial governments. In the city of Matanzas, eighty miles of streets were swept every day costing over $100,000 in 1899. In Cienfuegos, over fifty miles of city streets were swept daily. The seventy-eight members of the street-sweeping force in the city of Puerto Príncipe cleaned over twenty miles of streets at least five times a week and another nine miles of streets as needed at an average cost of nearly $100 a day. Even the three miles of streets in the town of Nuevitas were swept daily.[7] The U.S. occupation government also enacted regulations to keep the streets clean. In Puerto Príncipe, for example, residents who were found to have littered the street were fined two to four pesos.[8]

In Havana and its suburbs, the Department of Street Cleaning main-

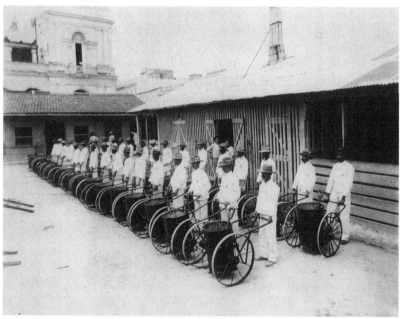

FIGURE 2 Street cleaning brigade in Havana, 1901. "Street Pickers with Can Carriers," File 1901/1652, Letters Received, 1899–1902, MGC/ RG 140

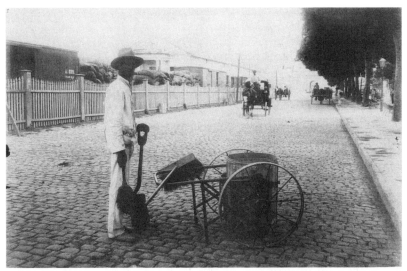

FIGURE 3 Street picker at work in Havana, 1901. "Picker with Outfit," File 1901/1652, Letters Received, 1899–1902, MGC/ RG 140

tained a force of over 500 inspectors, foremen, sweepers, and waterboys charged with the responsibility of sweeping 273 miles of streets every day. From July 1899 through February 1900, the expense for this work was reported to be nearly $150,000. During the second half of 1899, more than 55,000 tons of street refuse—an average of 299 tons each day—were collected and carted off.[9] To avoid disrupting traffic, the work was mostly done at night when the overnight teams would collect the sweepings and leave them in waste boxes. The next day, a force of "pickers," men equipped with a specially designed, two-wheeled iron can carrier, a broom, and a shovel, collected the sweepings. The pickers were also assigned routes along high traffic areas, "which they are expected to cover as many times during the day as may be necessary to keep the streets clean."[10]

In addition to being swept, Havana's streets were regularly doused with electrozone, a disinfectant manufactured through the electrolysis of seawater.[11] In July 1899, the Department of Engineers opened an electrozone plant in Havana that produced 24,000 gallons a day, about half of which was dedicated to street disinfection.[12] A force of mule-drawn sprinkling carts, each filled with up to 750 gallons of the liquid, covered Havana's streets once a day, and even more often in busy areas and districts where yellow fever was most prevalent.[13] By Febru-

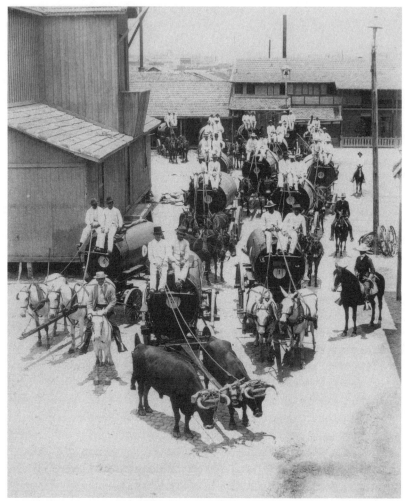

FIGURE 4 Electrozone sprinklers take to the streets of Havana, 1901. "Sprinklers Leaving the Yard. Stable No. 2," File 1901/1652, Letters Received, 1899–1902, MGC/ RG 140

ary 1901, Havana's sprinkling brigade had expanded to sixteen carts.[14] Other cities followed suit and established smaller sprinkling forces in the early months of the occupation.[15]

One of the first concerns when the U.S. Military Government took control of Cuba was that it needed to locate buildings for its headquarters and other government offices. This was not a straightforward task. Havana's chief engineer reported that the city's "public buildings were found in an exceedingly bad condition." Almost everything that could be removed—plumbing, fixtures, bathtubs, washstands, doors, and the like—had been sold off or destroyed. The buildings had to be cleaned and repaired "to remove all cause of infection" before the U.S. forces could occupy them.[16] The disinfecting work was extensive:

> [at] the commencement of the renovation of a building, disinfection was begun and was continued during the operation. Lime was used freely on all freshly excavated materials, and electrozone was sprayed with force pumps over every square inch of accessible area. Bichloride of mercury was used when the building had an unusually bad reputation. Walls and ceilings were thoroughly brushed, washed and scraped, floors scrubbed, walls kalsomined, and woodwork, doors and windows were repaired and painted. A great deal of plastering was found loose and replaced after thoroughly scraping the walls.[17]

Dozens of buildings in Havana received this treatment, including the military government's headquarters, the Military Governor's Palace, and the customs house. But the first building renovated was Las Ánimas, the city hospital dedicated by the occupation government to the treatment of yellow fever, indicating its high priority.[18]

The two major harbors of the island, Havana and Santiago, also received early attention as contributing to the environment that allowed yellow fever to thrive in Cuba. Even before the end of the war, Major General Leonard Wood, then commanding officer in Santiago, pointed out the need to clean the waterfront,

> which is, I believe, the focus of most of the fevers, and especially of the Yellow Fever in Santiago, as it is composed almost entirely of the washings of the city during the past three hundred years, and has formed a great mass of bank of corruption, which is exposed at low tide and must be most unhealthy and dangerous. It had been impossible to touch this during hot weather, as any stirring it up would result in an immediate outbreak of Yellow Fever; but this winter I intend to remove it with the use of suction dredges and scows and dump it way out to sea in deep water. This is going to cost a good deal, but it will result in the saving of life and greatly decrease the danger to our troops next summer.[19]

In Havana, a sewer emptying directly into the harbor had created particularly unsanitary conditions along the shore by the customs house.

As Havana's chief engineer reported, "a deposit of sewerage has been made, to so great an extent that at every landing of small boats the filth from the bottom is stirred up, and that there is in this angle a constant bubbling of the water, caused by the decomposition of material at the bottom, the whole being, in my judgment, very prejudicial to the health of the community."[20] In order to solve this problem, the Department of Engineers decided in August 1899 to extend the sewer pipe ten feet into the bay so that the current would carry the waste away from shore, then dredge the area of the customs house to remove the offensive material taking "all possible precautions by the use of disinfectants to remove danger of illness being caused by the work."[21]

Such precautions, however, did not assuage the fears of the commanding officer of the U.S. naval forces in Cuba, Rear Admiral B. J. Cromwell. Upon learning of the dredging operation, Cromwell charged to the waterfront and threatened to arrest anyone who continued the work. The following day he reported to General John Brooke, the island's military governor, what he saw as the problem:

> dredging was commenced, and continued for two hours after dark yesterday evening, and within forty yards of the Machina wharf, where the Marines are quartered and where one now lies sick with yellow fever. . . . The danger to the health from stirring, lifting and exposing the silt on the bottom of the Harbor at this season, and in the locality mentioned, is so manifest, that I hasten to acquaint you with the facts, that steps be taken to prevent a recurrence of the same.[22]

Other top officials agreed with Cromwell. Acting Chief Surgeon William Carter asked that the dredging be discontinued during the hot summer season: "We must assume that probably the most concentrated and potent Yellow fever infection is contained in the silt deposited near the shore in the vicinity of the Sewer opening and that the danger of infection is lessened by allowing this to remain under the surface during the hot season."[23]

Allowing this suspected concentration of yellow fever contamination to remain in the busy area of the customs house was not seen as a viable option. The work of dredging the harbor, Governor Brooke concluded, was being done with the greatest care and sanitary precautions. The dredging took place only at night. Before it began, one hundred pounds of chloride of lime were sprinkled in the bay over the part that was to be dredged that evening. On the wharf, electrozone was sprinkled over each bucket of material dumped. Halfway through the dredging process, another one hundred pounds of chloride of lime were sprinkled in the bay. Before six o'clock in the morning, the dredging was stopped, the dredge and wharf were scrubbed with electrozone, and the scows were cleaned and sprinkled with lime before the entire operation was anchored away from shore.[24] The engineers were sure that this process allowed the work to proceed while preventing any yellow fever threat.[25]

That same month, faced with yellow fever raging in Santiago de Cuba, General Wood, by then military governor of the Division of Santiago and Puerto Príncipe, ordered drastic measures: those without immunity to the disease were evacuated, and the city was put under strict quarantine. Only those who brought with them "a certificate that they have had yellow fever well pronounced . . . or certifying to ten years' continuous residence in Santiago" were permitted to disembark at the port.[26] U.S. soldiers and other government officials were moved to camps scattered from three to twenty miles from the city. The results of these steps were positive. Wood reported that the

> prompt disappearance of the disease as soon as our men were placed in camps on non-infected ground with plenty of space, sunlight and ventilation is suggestive of what we should do in the way of taking care of troops in Cuba and indicates clearly that these old towns should be avoided as much as possible as stations for our troops. . . . By observing this precaution and establishing our camps at an elevation upwards of 1000 feet, if possible, I believe we can count with almost absolute freedom from the disease.[27]

His recommendations were adopted: U.S. troops around the island were moved to camps at a distance from the towns for which they were responsible.

Quarantines were also imposed on places with yellow fever outbreaks. On September 20, 1899, after hearing about a "well authenticated case of yellow fever" in the town of Júcaro, the Júcaro and San Fernando Railroad Company immediately enacted new quarantine measures against the town. Printed in Spanish and in bold capital letters, notices announced that under no circumstance was anyone to be transported from Júcaro to Ciego de Ávila on the railroad, no employee of the railroad would leave the train while in Júcaro or come into contact with anyone there, that the train would be allowed to stay there no more than fifteen minutes, and that no merchandise from Júcaro would be taken onboard.[28] The U.S. Marine Hospital Service (USMHS) established inspection stations at ten Cuban ports to prevent intraisland shipping from spreading infection: due to yellow fever epidemics, all baggage from Santiago de Cuba, Guantánamo, Baoquirí, Nuevitas, and Gibara was inspected and, if needed, disinfected to destroy the suspected yellow fever germs. Only passengers immune to yellow fever were permitted to travel from these ports.[29]

Ships arriving from foreign ports with suspected cases of yellow fever were forced to anchor miles from shore and remain under quarantine for five days before being allowed to dock and unload.[30] Passengers arriving from locations known to have yellow fever, such as the Mexican ports of Veracruz and Progreso, were required to have their baggage disinfected upon arrival. Their trunks and bags were taken away, opened, and emptied. The contents were then placed in wire baskets that were then dipped in formaldehyde, a process no germ would survive. After this procedure, they were repacked, labeled "Disinfected and Passed," and made available for retrieval.[31]

Quarantine measures extended even to the handling of mail. When, in July 1899, the chief surgeon of the Department of Matanzas and Santa Clara recommended to the postal authorities of that department that they disinfect all mail coming from Manzanillo, Santiago de Cuba, and Puerto Príncipe on account of yellow fever in those cities, he was surprised to learn that all of Santiago's outgoing mail was already being disinfected.[32]

The plans to control yellow fever were not only aimed at protecting the island from another outbreak, but also to make sure that the disease did not make it to ports in the United States and become epidemic. For this reason, the occupation's early steps against yellow fever also included new regulations for baggage shipped from Cuba to ports in the United States. These new rules required that all baggage or personal effects bound for points in the U.S. South—as far north as the southern boundary of Maryland—were to be disinfected and labeled before being allowed to leave the island. Bags destined for ports north of Maryland's southern border were inspected and then disinfected only when deemed necessary.[33]

At the end of 1899, these early efforts appeared to have met with some success. The year had been a relatively mild one with respect to yellow fever in Cuba, particularly in Havana, where the disease caused only 103 deaths, the fewest on record.[34] But with the completion of the

Spanish evacuation and with the U.S. authorities settled in, the occupation government intensified its efforts against the disease.

Cuba's new military governor, Major General Leonard Wood, was
well prepared for the task of battling yellow fever when he took charge in
late December 1899. He had earned a medical degree from Harvard and
served as an army surgeon before switching to the command ranks during the western campaigns against the Apache in the late 1880s and then
serving as the commanding officer of the 1st U.S. Volunteer Cavalry—
the Rough Riders—during the war against the Spanish in Cuba. As
governor of the Division of Santiago and Puerto Príncipe, his policy of
relocating troops and other nonimmunes had successfully stifled the yellow fever epidemic in the city of Santiago de Cuba. Havana's new chief
sanitary officer was similarly well-qualified. As an army surgeon, Major
William C. Gorgas had spent years combating yellow fever epidemics in
Texas and Florida before being transferred to Havana in January 1899
to ready Las Ánimas to serve as the city's yellow fever hospital.[35]

Gorgas began his thorough reorganization of the health department
in regards to yellow fever by creating a systematized process of reporting the disease in Havana. Suspected cases were forwarded to the Board
of Physicians, which later became the Yellow Fever Commission. After
visiting and investigating the cases, the commission would present case
reports to the adjutant general of the Division of Cuba, in the office of
the governor. Additionally, the reports were forwarded to the island's
chief surgeon, the Havana newspaper *La Lucha,* the Health Office of
Florida, and a representative of the Associated Press.[36] By Governor
Wood's order, the cooperation of Cuban physicians was mandatory under the threat of "a severe penalty for non-compliance."[37]

Upon being diagnosed with yellow fever, patients were immediately
removed to the yellow fever wing of the local infectious and contagious
disease facility in Havana, Las Ánimas Hospital. There they were kept
in strict isolation. The stringent procedures were enacted in hospitals
throughout the island. When an army private escaped from the yellow
fever wing of the Military Hospital of Matanzas, everyone who came
into contact with him was disinfected and detained under observation
for four days. Even when the private later died and the doctors dis-
agreed on whether the cause of his death had indeed been yellow fever,
the small possibility that it could have been yellow fever was considered
sufficient to warrant an order that no one attend his funeral except the
ceremonial firing squad.[38]

When a patient was confirmed to be suffering from yellow fever, the authorities would immediately act to address the location of infection. The process of disinfecting began at the place of residence. During the investigation of the cases "an agent of the Sanitary Department was stationed at the door, and the apartments inspected several times a day by a superior officer to see that the quarantine and proper hygienic precautions were carried out."[39] Once the patient was removed from the home, and the furniture taken to be disinfected at the facilities of the Marine Hospital Service,[40] the contaminated room, as well as those connected to it, were disinfected by blasting every surface with a solution of bichloride of mercury. In another room, hooks were driven into the walls and rope strung from one to the other, creating a place for all of the fabrics in the apartment to be hung. Sanitation workers then closed this room, sealed off all of its cracks, and filled it with formaldehyde gas. The rest of the rooms in the house were then fumigated.[41] Often the bedding and clothing of yellow fever patients were burned. Although this caused considerable hardship to impoverished victims of yellow fever, requests for reimbursement were summarily denied on the grounds that the authorities' actions were necessary to prevent contagion.[42] After this process was complete, a squad was sent to pick up the disposed materials from the disinfected house. The owner of the house was then ordered to make repairs and sanitary renovations as deemed necessary. One week later, inspectors visited the house to ensure compliance. Any failure to complete the ordered work resulted in a fine of ten dollars that was turned over to a judge to collect, and under the supervision of the chief of police, the house was closed until the sanitary work was completed.[43] Usually the fines were imposed for the purpose of compelling compliance and were often dropped for owners who promptly acted on orders.[44] In extreme cases, such as the building of the newspaper *Diario de la Marina*, the site of seven yellow fever cases between September 1899 and May 1900, orders were issued barring nonimmune persons from living in the building.[45]

Even rumors of yellow fever incited a quick response. When Governor Wood received a letter complaining that a young girl whose parents had died of yellow fever was going door to door in Havana looking for a job and thereby exposing others to the disease, inspectors were sent immediately to investigate the possibility that such a potentially infected person was wandering the streets. In less than twenty-four hours a report on the situation was complete. The inspector found that the address the girl reportedly provided as her previous residence did not exist, but no one on the street had died of yellow fever, and the only death in the neighborhood was a woman who lived in a tenement house. When the inspector arrived at the tenement, he found the disinfecting brigade already at work. The woman, it turned out, had died of tuberculosis.[46] There was a sense of relief that it was merely tuberculosis instead of the dreaded yellow fever. Whereas Cubans were more afflicted by tuberculosis than any other disease, that was not a priority for the U.S. sanitary authorities. Yellow fever, on the other hand, elicited an instant response.

But the Sanitary Department of the occupation government did not wait for reports of yellow fever to take action against the disease. Houses in Havana were inspected three times a year. In order to accomplish this feat, the city was divided into twenty inspection districts, each with a chief inspector who every day received orders to report on certain residences. Inspectors then issued orders to the owners to clean their homes, whitewash with lime, make plumbing repairs, or take any other measures deemed necessary to sanitize their property. A week after an initial order was issued, the house was reinspected. If the work ordered had not been started, the homeowner was warned that if the work was not begun promptly a fine would be issued. A week later, the inspector visited the house again, and if the work was still not begun, legal proceedings to collect the fine were initiated. If the fine was ignored and the work still not done, the city completed the work and billed the owner for the expense. "In cases that are pressing, such as unusually dirty tenement houses, or similar places, the department puts in its own force and thoroughly cleans and disinfects the premises. For this purpose we have a force of sixty men, divided into two squads, under the charge of inspectors and foremen; besides smaller squads for two of the suburban towns [Regla and Guanabacoa]."[47] In some cases elsewhere on the island, extremely dirty buildings were simply demolished.[48] A record on every house in the city was kept in Gorgas's offices.[49]

The authorities also targeted filth below ground as a source of infection. In Havana, Santiago de Cuba, and other major cities, there were no general systems of sewers; the vast majority of buildings had their own cesspools to deal with the disposal of sewage. To avoid the threat of infection, these cesspools had to be maintained in a sanitary condition and cleaned periodically. When sanitary inspectors encountered a problem, they referred the case to the Night Soil Department of the Department of Engineers, which emptied and sanitized the cities' cesspools. Sanitary inspectors and engineers noted that most cesspools in the cities had not been properly maintained for decades. "In many cases, where the parties were poor, proper closets and vaults were constructed where none had existed previously. In many cases, on the other hand, five or six vaults were found beneath the patios which had to be pumped out, disinfected and sealed."[50] Even with the system of inspection and sanitation of cesspools in place, the disposal of sewage was considered a serious threat to the occupation government's fight against yellow fever. As Gorgas wrote in November 1900, "I do not believe that our present system of disinfection and isolation will answer in itself to eradicate yellow fever from Havana, but must be supplemented by a general sewerage system, and I earnestly urge that this be commenced at the earliest possible date."[51]

Governor Wood's earlier experience with the yellow fever epidemic in Santiago de Cuba demonstrated that, when sanitation efforts failed, the spread of yellow fever could be stopped by removing nonimmune people from any potential source of infection. Therefore, nonimmune camps were established outside of towns where yellow fever was epidemic and nonimmunes from those towns were forced to move into them. Places where people congregated, such as saloons and cafes, were also ordered closed in these towns.[52] U.S. health authorities performed inspections and reported not only any suspicion of yellow fever, but also any nonimmunes living in quarantined areas in violation of the law.[53] The sanitary officer of the towns had to report by nine in the morning daily to the chief surgeon of the province the names of the people in the camp along with the specific location of their recent residences. Nonimmune people were to remain in the camps at least fifteen days after which, if they did not have a fever, they were given health certificates from both the chief surgeon of the department and the Marine Hospital Service and could leave with their disinfected belongings.[54]

The removal of the entire nonimmune population from Havana was considered impossible, but some steps could be taken to limit the spread of yellow fever.[55] During the occupation, U.S. authorities encouraged the immigration of Spanish farm workers to work the fields in Cuba. This was due to the fact that during the Cuban war for independence, both the insurgents and the Spanish army sought to deprive their opponents of resources by destroying the rural economy. The Cuban rebels burned the crops of landowners who failed to "contribute" to the cause; the Spanish ruined the plantations of those who did. Under General Valeriano Weyler, the Spanish army sought to relocate the entire rural population to concentration camps in the outskirts of Cuba's cities, where they could be easily monitored and unable to support the insurgents. These *reconcentrados* had little access to food or clean water, and the camps were soon wracked with disease. By 1897, when the reconcentration policy was abandoned after much local and international criticism, over

200,000 people had already perished in the camps. When the United States assumed control, the devastation of the Cuban countryside presented attractive opportunities to U.S. investors. But reestablishing the island's sugar industry and its other agricultural operations would require a new rural workforce—and that workforce would have to remain free of yellow fever.

The trickle of Spanish immigrants that began in 1899 soon became a flood: in the first week of October 1900, close to 3,000 immigrants arrived in Havana, compared with 2,248 for the entire month in 1899.[56] Many of these new arrivals fell victim to yellow fever before they could move on to jobs in the countryside.[57] Even though the sanitation of Havana was improving, Gorgas concluded that yellow fever would worsen as the city's population of nonimmunes increased: "My impression is that since September to the present time the rate of immigration has been four or five times as large as normal. This difference is the cause for the increase in yellow fever between this June and last. If we had no non-immunes, we would have no yellow fever."[58]

The immigrants from Spain invited after the war by the U.S. occupation government to help repopulate the island's interior were vulnerable to yellow fever only if they lingered in Havana. This danger, like that to soldiers, was quite easily averted once it was identified. The new arrivals would not be permitted even to pass through Havana. Gorgas proposed the creation of an immigrant detention camp outside the city: "The idea being to collect all the immigrants and take them right from the shipping to this settlement, without coming near the City of Havana, and then distribute them to their various destinations around the island."[59] The immigrants, he argued, "would be very much better off than if allowed to come into the city, and certainly very much less likely to contract Yellow Fever."[60] A board of medical officers, convened to discuss and advise on the feasibility and benefits of a detention camp for immigrants, concluded that the camp would not only "avoid the spread of yellow fever" in Havana but also would prevent the immigrants from "living or working in any infected or suspicious place and also any agglomeration or crowding of non-immunes any where."[61] The camp was opened in November 1900. When Spanish immigrants arrived in Havana, they were taken to the camp immediately after the ship was inspected, and they remained there until they found employment in the countryside.[62]

This logic also applied to the officials of the occupation government. When several government buildings in Havana were reinspected and found to be threatened by yellow fever, they were quarantined for disinfection. The offices were then relocated to nearby towns or to military camps. The commanders of these camps took care to isolate the officials and employees coming from Havana before allowing them to enter the camp.[63] Even after the buildings were again considered sanitary, the people working in them were not completely free from the possibility of catching yellow fever after work. To mitigate this threat, all the clerks and employees who worked at headquarters buildings were "permitted and advised to seek lodging in the country, preferably at Vedado and Guanabacoa," and allowed to leave work early enough to get home before dark.[64]

Although the U.S. authorities had taken steps to protect against the introduction of yellow fever from outside the island early in the occupation, these measures were expanded and standardized in the fall of 1900. On September 28, 1900, Governor Wood promulgated new laws stating that all ships, regardless of whether there was a diseased person on board, entering into port must immediately hoist a yellow flag—the "yellow jack"—to indicate that the ship had not yet been inspected. All passengers were then required to go on deck for inspection by a sanitary inspector from the USMHS. Only after the inspection was complete and the flag lowered was anyone permitted to leave the ship. Passengers' baggage was then inspected and, when deemed necessary, disinfected.[65]

Additional quarantine measures were adopted as well. The director of general sanitation in Cienfuegos requested an order that "all passengers proceeding from Havana may not be allowed to embark for Cienfuegos without being first fumigated with their baggage, and that all acclimated foreigners besides being subject to these measures, should bring a certificate of acclimation of the epidemic which occupies us."[66] The USMHS further recommended that at Cienfuegos, all nonimmunes "should be kept under daily observation reporting to the local health officers once a day for the period of five days and their baggage disinfected" with the help of the quarantine officers from nearby seaport towns.[67]

Resistance to and Acceptance of Colonial Public Health

This thorough but burdensome inspection and sanitation regime prompted a variety of responses. Gorgas later recounted the reaction of one Cuban woman to the disinfection of her home. He visited the tenement house when the disinfection brigade was at work and the residents waited in the patio sitting with all their belongings "in the most uncomfortable and disconsolate way." When asked what was going on by her husband who had just arrived at the scene, the woman, according to Gorgas, replied " that she did not know, but that it was 'just one of the ways of those crazy Americans.' Her good nature made quite an impression upon me. She evidently had no particular sympathy with what we were doing, but had the general idea that we were trying to do it for their good, notwithstanding that she considered it as one of our extreme and crazy ideas."[68]

Others were less sympathetic. Investigators in the city of Quemados, in Pinar del Río, ordered a group of Syrians living in a tenement house to leave their homes so that the cleaning brigade could proceed with the disinfection of the building. The Syrians misunderstood the order and, believing that they were being deported from the province, protested furiously.[69] In Havana, after a thorough inspection and subsequent orders and reinspections of his house, accompanied by the threat that the house would be boarded up, one homeowner complained that while the order by the Sanitary Department to whitewash the house with lime was being completed, he did not think that the department had any right to order the changing of the floors. "It seems to me that the Sanitary department is carrying things too far and is often annoying the inhabitants of this city with their orders," he complained to Governor Wood's office. "I could tell you of many cases where the Sanitary Dept is abusing the pacific people of Havana."[70] But all such complaints fell on deaf ears; the ordered work was completed.

Why did the extensive and intrusive sanitation measures against yellow fever not provoke greater resistance among the Cubans? Disease and the public-health responses to it have often touched off violence in other colonial settings. But several factors affect the extent of resistance engendered by epidemic disease and colonial public-health efforts. The first of these factors are the characteristics of the disease, in particular, its place of origin and its pattern of infection. In places where epidemics were brought by the colonizers and disproportionately afflicted indigenous populations, they were more likely to stoke conflict than where the disease was of native origin and ravaged occupier and occupied alike. When the New World smallpox pandemic reached northeastern Brazil in 1562, the disease triggered an indigenous resistance movement dedicated to exterminating the Portuguese colonists who had brought the disease; the movement remained a force in the region for decades.[71] Similarly, cholera brought to North American Plains Indians by passing settlers in the mid-nineteenth century sparked an upsurge in violence as the disease "hardened nomadic tribes' attitudes toward whites and left them more willing to retaliate."[72]

Conflicting cultural understandings of disease and medicine also contributed to resistance to colonial public health measures. When bubonic plague reached Bombay in 1896, British officials adopted a wide range of aggressive measures across India to protect trade, including a massive sanitation campaign, the prohibition of pilgrimages, and the forced hospitalization of all plague cases. This last provision—which removed Indians (and most distressingly, Indian women) from the loving care of their families to what they viewed as "a place of pollution, contaminated by blood and feces, inimical to caste, religion, and purdah"— repeatedly incited riots in Bombay. Other insensitive steps also resulted in sporadic violence, including the assassination of the chairman of the Plague Committee in the restive city of Pune.[73] But where native medical traditions were more pluralistic and colonial public health could be adapted to indigenous traditions, as was the case in Yunnan, the French sphere of influence in southwestern China, measures to prevent the spread of epidemic disease were readily accepted.[74]

These factors all worked against extreme resistance in Cuba. Yellow fever was endemic in Havana, and it only afflicted newcomers. Cubans therefore did not see the disease as a form of attack to be resisted. Further, unlike some other colonial situations, Cuban and U.S. physicians shared the same medical-cultural tradition. By the end of the nineteenth century most Cuban doctors were trained primarily in the United States, so the yellow fever elimination efforts in Cuba were not the focus of clashing medical knowledge between the colonizer and the colonized. Therefore, it is not surprising that, in relation to yellow fever under the U.S. occupation, resistance to sanitary reforms was minimal, with a few scattered complaints and no upsurge in violent confrontation.

Why Focus on Yellow Fever?

All the cleaning, sweeping, planning, disinfecting, and quarantining by the U.S. occupation government centered around yellow fever. There are several possible explanations for the rigorous attention the disease received in Cuba. Some authors have suggested that the U.S. authorities were interested in yellow fever in order to protect the troops stationed on the island. Others, consistent with the portrayal of the U.S. occupation of the island as a humanitarian effort, have presented the concern with yellow fever as an attempt by the United States to improve the health of the Cuban people. The evidence does not support these accounts. Instead, the records show that, as an exercise in colonial public health, these exertions were primarily motivated by the U.S. government's long-standing concern with the threat that yellow fever in Cuba posed to the economy of the U.S. South through trade.

The focus on combating yellow fever during the U.S. occupation of Cuba is often argued to have been an effort to protect the U.S. troops still stationed throughout the island.[75] Although a yellow fever outbreak among the troops was a constant worry of U.S. military officers in the course of the war, after the fighting was over U.S. soldiers could be and were purposefully isolated from the urban populations where yellow fever was most likely to strike. Yellow fever in Cuba was almost exclusively an urban disease, concentrated in Havana with some cases occurring in Santiago de Cuba and other cities and towns. As described above, the U.S. troops were transferred to camps outside the cities after the war. The success of this simple measure meant that during the occupation, malaria was a much more serious problem within the ranks than yellow fever. For example, each of the 2,146 U.S. soldiers stationed in Santiago suffered from an average of two cases of malaria from July 1899 to June 1900, but, even in Havana, there were few cases of yellow fever: there were only twenty-four cases and seven deaths of yellow fever among all the troops in Havana in 1900.[76] Gorgas wrote, "at Havana a greater number of persons died from malaria every year than from yellow fever [but] all our efforts and attention were given to the eradication of yellow fever."[77] If the occupation government's primary concerns were for the health of the U.S. soldiers, it would have focused its attention on malaria rather than yellow fever.

Other scholars have argued that the occupation was a benevolent gesture on the part of the United States toward the Cuban people.[78] The sanitation efforts have been explained as "absolutely essential to build[ing] an independent republic whose people could be free of the fetters of poverty and sickness."[79] There is little support, however, for this position with respect to the occupation government's war against yellow fever. Most Cubans did not believe that they were at risk for the disease; the conventional wisdom held that Cubans were immune to it. Yellow fever, although terrible and often fatal to adults, causes such mild symptoms in children that infection most often goes unnoticed. Further, a single bout of the disease generates a permanent immunity. Together, these two aspects made it of little concern to lifelong inhabitants of areas where yellow fever was endemic or frequently epidemic: nearly all had become immune to the disease through childhood infection. Cubans, while making up the largest share of Havana's population, were the least affected group in the city. In addition, mortuary statistics demonstrate that while the occupation government was focusing its ef-

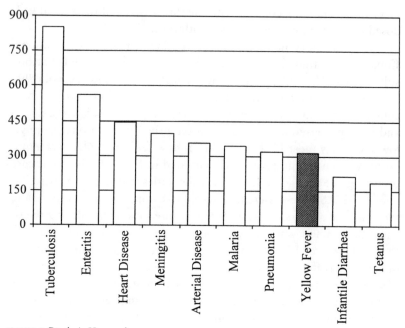

FIGURE 5 Deaths in Havana, by cause, 1900

forts on yellow fever, more Cubans were killed by tuberculosis than any other disease—a fact well known to the U.S. authorities: "tuberculosis is always present, and claims more victims annually than any other fever; yet it is not feared and receives little attention," the USMHS reported.[80] Indeed, many diseases caused more suffering to Cubans than yellow fever. In Havana during 1900, "yellow fever stands eighth in the records of deaths for the year. Tuberculosis with 851 deaths, diarrhoea and enteritis with 506 deaths, organic diseases of the heart with 443 deaths, meningitis with 395 deaths, diseases of the arteries with 357 deaths, malaria with 344 deaths and pneumonia with 319 deaths, each have caused a greater mortality than yellow fever."[81] The occupation government's single-minded determination to eliminate yellow fever, then, was only secondarily motivated by a concern for the health of Cubans or for the health of the U.S. troops.

Although preserving the health of the occupation troops and administrators as well as that of the local workforce were among the concerns of U.S. public health officials, what *most* concerned the occupation government about yellow fever in Cuba was its ability to spread along the arteries of trade and so threaten the economy of the U.S. South. Governor Wood commented privately to Secretary of War Elihu Root that if tariffs were raised for Cuban tobacco and sugar: "In the first place, one of the great purposes of our intervention will not have been realized ... the old unsanitary conditions will quickly return; conditions of yellow fever which it is estimated cost our Southern States in injury to commerce and cost to quarantine not less than from forty to fifty million dollars per year."[82] Gorgas later explained that,

> We had believed, for a generation or two, that if, in any way, we could get rid of yellow fever in Havana, yellow fever would cease to be a menace to our Southern states. So that practically, the sanitation of Cuba centered about the sanitation of Havana; and the sanitation of Havana, in our mind, consisted almost entirely of the sanitation with regard to yellow fever. We then believed that, if any disease was caused by filth, yellow fever was that disease; and all our thoughts, and all our efforts, were centered about cleaning up.[83]

The U.S. war on yellow fever, then, was *not* principally aimed at protecting the occupying force or improving the health of Cubans. It was above all an attempt to eliminate the source of the infection that had ground the economy of the Mississippi Valley to a halt in 1878 and burdened southern trade and commerce ever since.

By the end of 1900, however, it had become clear that the occupation government's attempts to eliminate the threat to the U.S. South of yellow fever in Cuba by cleaning up the island had failed. Despite the city's extensive sanitation program, the number of deaths from yellow fever in Havana had tripled from the previous year, and yellow fever cases had increased by over 350 percent. Figure 6 illustrates the severity of Havana's 1900 yellow fever season compared with the previous year.[84]

The sharp increase in yellow fever did not go unnoticed in the United States. North American newspapers repeatedly accused the occupation government of neglecting its duty to stop the disease.[85] The government was quick to counter these claims, pointing to the much-improved sanitary conditions of Havana.[86] But there was no denying that the disease was striking even high-ranking occupation officials—those "whose surroundings were the best and as good as it was possible to make them."[87] Practically the entire staff of the Office of the Collector of Customs in the Port of Santiago had been taken sick with yellow fever in the span of two weeks in August 1899, paralyzing the work of that office.[88] The death of Major Watt Peterson in October 1900 was widely reported, including in the *New York Tribune* and the *Atlanta Constitution*.[89] As

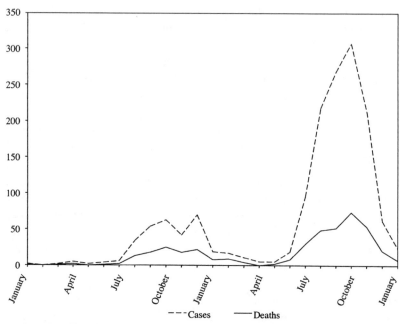

FIGURE 6 Monthly yellow fever cases and deaths in Havana, January 1899 to January 1901

Gorgas later recalled, "Our sanitary measures, if they had any effect upon yellow fever, seemed to increase it. The cleanest and best built part of the city seemed to suffer most from the disease, and the best fed and best cared for part of the population was that which had the largest rate of yellow fever."[90]

Governor Wood had held the same suspicions during his time in Santiago: yellow fever seemed to strike without regard to sanitary precautions. The outbreak in Santiago de Cuba was initially thought to result from the digging involved in paving and laying water pipes in the city's streets, but those who worked in these endeavors were not affected as much as other nonimmunes within the city. "The medical fraternity are inclined to attribute the outbreak to the unusually hot and dry weather, but candidly no one seems to be able to give a satisfactory explanation as to its causes. This is accounted for by the fact that very little is known about the cause of yellow fever," he wrote.[91] The worsening of the disease in 1900 reinforced his doubts: "This year, strange enough, the fever has cropped up in some little towns in the interior, like Santa Clara, in buildings where troops lived all last year without a case. The house in which poor Edmunds got the fever was occupied all last Summer and Winter by Dr. Kaine's family, including his wife and little children. In other words there is a good deal about this disease which we do not understand."[92]

To eliminate the disease that threatened the economy of the entire U.S. South, the occupation government had taken every step suggested by current medical knowledge, no matter how difficult, from searching every house in Havana for unsanitary conditions once every four months to relocating the nonimmune populations of towns across the island. No effort had been spared, but by the end of 1900, the "great object" of the occupation appeared no closer to being accomplished than it had in 1898.

4

The Hunt for the Mosquito

"If," says Dr. Horlbeck, "the mosquito is the true vehicle of communication, it at once simplifies a most important matter, perhaps the most important matter affecting the health and well-being for six months of at least 10,000,000 people living in the South." . . . If the Finlay theory is true, the sufferer from abroad can be made harmless at the cost of a few yards of mosquito netting. He may die himself, but he will not kill others and he will not interrupt the business of railways or steamboats.　　　　　**New York Times, November 10, 1900**

: : :

After two years of intense efforts aimed at controlling yellow fever, in 1900 the number of cases began to increase again. Despite the determination of U.S. authorities to sanitize Havana and force its citizens to maintain clean households, yellow fever was again ravaging the city and putting at risk the growing economic interaction between Cuba and the United States. The quarantines and extensive disinfection routines that were established to protect ports across the U.S. South from the spread of yellow fever restricted the trade and the economic exchange between the two countries.

This chapter traces the history of the theory that linked yellow fever with the mosquito, its confirmation, and its application to the efforts against yellow fever in Cuba. The focus of much contemporary medical research was on the relation between bacteria and disease, and the early work of a U.S. commission sent to Cuba in 1900 centered on a bacteriological theory of yellow fever. The commission, however, eventually took up and confirmed the theory of a Cuban doctor that the disease was carried by a species of mosquito and not by filth. This confirmation led to a reassessment of existing policies against yellow fever. Although it maintained its campaign for cleanliness, the U.S. occupation government reorganized its sanitation force to focus primarily on the destruction of mosquito breeding places and the isolation of yellow fever patients from mosquitoes. Although many Cubans—and many U.S. officials— were skeptical of the new antimosquito efforts, the policies of the military government succeeded in ridding Cuba of yellow fever.

The Mosquito Theory of Yellow Fever:
Finlay, Carter, Lazear, and Reed

The story of how Carlos Finlay identified and the U.S. Yellow Fever Commission headed by Walter Reed confirmed the mosquito vector of yellow fever has often been told, but the facts have remained sharply disputed. Some historians give Finlay all of the credit for the discovery, arguing that Reed merely gained broad acceptance for work completed by the Cuban doctor.[1] Others laud Reed as the brilliant scientist singlehandedly responsible for the advance, marginalizing Finlay or even omitting him from the tale entirely.[2]

The very importance of the breakthrough is likely the ultimate source of the discrepancies and confusion. Not surprisingly, many who participated in the events afterwards embellished their roles for the sake of fame, professional advancement, or other rewards; too often, later writers unquestioningly accepted these self-serving statements as true. National pride sometimes also played a role, as both U.S. and Cuban authors extolled the contributions of their countrymen and minimized those of others, a point examined in greater detail in a later chapter. Enduring interest in the episode compounded both of these problems, as subsequent authors uncritically echoed earlier works.

As is often true of great discoveries, many people made important contributions to the mosquito theory of yellow fever and its confirmation. Finlay did correctly identify the species of mosquito that carries yellow fever, and Reed did design and carry out the careful experiments that convincingly demonstrated that the bite of this mosquito does transmit the disease and that the filth of yellow fever patients does not. But Finlay did not realize that a mosquito does not become infectious immediately after biting a yellow fever patient. Henry Rose Carter established the crucial detail that the disease requires nearly two weeks of extrinsic incubation. And it was not Reed, but Jesse Lazear, a member of the U.S. commission who, tired of his superior's obsession with bacteria, decided to begin experiments with mosquitoes that took Carter's discovery into account. Only after Lazear became the first to succeed in experimentally inducing yellow fever—and died in a later effort—did Reed take up the mosquito theory.

: : :

By the time of the U.S. occupation of Cuba, Carlos J. Finlay had been studying yellow fever in Havana for more than twenty years. A Cuban physician, Finlay had been a member of the Auxiliary Spanish Commission to the 1879 Havana Yellow Fever Commission organized by the U.S. National Board of Health. In the aftermath of the devastating 1878 Mississippi Valley epidemic, the commission had visited Havana to study various aspects of the disease. First, it sought to ascertain the sanitary condition of ports, particularly Havana and Matanzas, to make these places more hygienic and thus prevent yellow fever from reaching ships and spreading to the United States. Second, it sought to study the pathology of yellow fever, to determine its symptoms and how it progressed once in the human body. Finally, the commission sought to verify that yellow fever was endemic to Havana.[3] While in Cuba, the commission obtained assistance from local physicians, including Finlay. After the U.S. doctors departed, Finlay continued to investigate how yellow fever was spread.

In 1881, Finlay presented a new hypothesis on the propagation of yellow fever to the Academy of Sciences of Havana.[4] The most distinctive symptom of the disease was hemorrhage, particularly of the gums, nose, and stomach; yellow fever was often called *vómito negro* (black vomit) because those who suffered severe cases of the disease vomited congealed blood. As the disease seemed to attack principally blood and blood vessels, it had to be transported from the bloodstream of one person to another by something—something, Finlay surmised, like a blood-sucking insect.[5]

The mosquito was the prime candidate. Not only do mosquitoes feed on blood, Finlay observed, but their behavior also exhibits several similarities to that of yellow fever. Mosquitoes are not found in high elevations; neither were yellow fever epidemics. Mosquitoes and yellow fever cases both dwindled in the winter months. Mosquitoes do not ordinarily travel great distances on their own, but they can be transported. Yellow fever cases typically concentrated in a single location but could also jump erratically, even over long distances. He settled on a small, striped-and-spotted, house-dwelling variety—the mosquito that would eventually become known as *aedes aegypti*—as the most likely suspect.

On this basis, Finlay hypothesized that three conditions were necessary for the spread of yellow fever. First, a mosquito must bite a yellow fever patient; second, it had to survive to bite again; and third, the mosquito had to bite a nonimmune person. "I believe that, in Havana, the three conditions above mentioned have always coincided in the years of most marked yellow fever mortality," Finlay offered.[6] He then described an experiment in which he had captured a mosquito, allowed it to bite a yellow fever patient, and then allowed it to bite a nonimmune research subject. Three out of four inoculations completed at the time of the presentation had resulted in mild cases of yellow fever, Finlay claimed; the fourth one was then still within the incubation period of the disease.

Although Finlay's theory and his subsequent articles were circulated in academic and medical circles around the world over the next two decades, his experiments were scrutinized and discarded as unreliable. Some historians have argued that the reason for the widespread dismissal of Finlay's theory was that U.S. sanitarians viewed Cubans, and Latin Americans for that matter, as inferior and Latin American scientists as incompetent. At the time, however, the principal objection to his work was that his experiments were conducted in Havana, where yellow fever was endemic; his nonimmune research subjects, critics suggested, could have been infected with yellow fever through exposure to the contaminated city rather than by the mosquito bites administered by Finlay.[7]

So in late June 1900, with the campaign against yellow fever in Cuba foundering, the surgeon general of the U.S. Army, George M. Sternberg, created a yellow fever commission to investigate the cause of yellow fever. It has been assumed that the reason the commission was created was because Cuba offered the perfect opportunity for U.S. scientists to study yellow fever in its endemic form.[8] But in reality, it was the failure of traditional methods of combating the disease that spurred its creation. Headed by Walter Reed and composed of physicians Jesse Lazear, James Carroll, and Arístides Agramonte, the commission was based at Columbia Barracks, in Quemados, a place known to be free of yellow fever. Sternberg, a former member of the 1879 Havana Yellow Fever Commission, asked Reed to investigate the claims of the Italian bacteriologist Giuseppe Sanarelli, who in 1897 had linked yellow fever to a bacteria, *bacillus icteroides*. The apparent failure of the campaign by the occupation government to control yellow fever through sanitation made further investigation of the cause of the disease necessary, but it also provided an ideal opportunity to study Sanarelli's bacillus. Indeed, several of the commission's members had already been working in Cuba on the causes of yellow fever; Lazear had been at Columbia Barracks for months investigating the etiology of yellow fever when Walter Reed arrived. Agramonte, a Havana physician who had found Sanarelli's bacillus in autopsies of yellow fever patients during the yellow fever epidemic in Santiago in 1898, had continued his studies of the disease.

The commission's initial experiments consisted of drawing the blood of yellow fever patients and examining it for bacteria. In the eighteen cases examined, however, none of the blood cultures showed signs of Sanarelli's bacillus. In addition, none of the bacillus was found in eleven autopsies of yellow fever patients.[9] There was no evidence in these experiments that Sanarelli's bacillus was in any way related to yellow fever. By mid-July 1900, Lazear was convinced that the cause of yellow fever lay elsewhere, but Reed and Carroll remained focused on the bacteriological research.[10] After Lazear's death, Reed would insist that he directed all of Lazear's work, a claim that was echoed by Reed's biographers and by later scholars.[11] But the shift in focus away from the study of bacteria was made by Lazear, who, while the head of the commission was not paying attention, took the opportunity to explore a different theory of transmission.

Lazear's conversations with Dr. Henry Rose Carter, of the U.S. Marine Hospital Service (USMHS), pointed his work in a new direction. Before being stationed in Havana, Carter had studied yellow fever epidemics in the U.S. South. His work on the 1898 epidemic in the towns of Orwood and Taylor, Mississippi, demonstrated that there was a lag of two to three weeks between the first case of yellow fever and any subsequent cases in the same location.[12] Carter believed that this lapse of time could be due to an intermediate host, providing some support for Finlay's mosquito theory. In his experiments, however, Finlay had never waited more than a few days before allowing an infected mosquito to bite his research subject, not long enough according to Carter's findings. In June 1900, Carter had sent Lazear an article he published on the Mississippi towns with a note attached:

> I think that this is about the argument I made to you yesterday
> and which you can, naturally, examine better when written out.
> As I said; to me the a-priori argument for Dr. F's theory has

much in its favor and to me is more than plausible, although his observations as I read them are not convincing, scarcely corroborative.[13]

In August, Lazear began experiments to test whether mosquitoes could convey yellow fever. He raised mosquitoes from eggs provided by Finlay, allowed them to bite yellow fever patients, and then allowed them to bite nonimmune subjects, including himself. He carefully recorded both how long the yellow fever patient had been suffering before being bitten and the time that elapsed before the subject was bitten. Lazear's first nine trials, conducted between August 11 and 25, replicated the Finlay experiments: the interval between the bite of the patient and that of the subject was relatively short, and none of the subjects developed yellow fever.[14] But his colleagues paid little attention to this work. Reed, in fact, had left Cuba for a two-month trip to Washington on August 2.[15] Both Reed and Carroll, Lazear complained in a letter to his wife on August 23, "are interested in the controversy with Sanarelli, and they think about that all the time."[16] That would soon change.

On August 27, Lazear persuaded Carroll to submit to bites from four infected mosquitoes. Although three of the mosquitoes had bitten yellow fever patients less than a week before, the fourth had been infected twelve days earlier. Four days later, Carroll realized he had a fever, but he gave so little importance to Lazear's work that he first tested himself for malaria.[17] That afternoon he was bedridden, and the next day he was diagnosed with a severe case of yellow fever. A week later, after hearing of the events in Cuba and of Carroll's subsequent recovery, Reed wrote from Washington congratulating his friend on his survival. As a postscript, he asked incredulously, "Did the *mosquito do it?*"[18]

Lazear had already initiated a more carefully controlled attempt to find out. On August 31, the same day that Carroll fell sick, Lazear administered a series of mosquito bites to William H. Dean, a U.S. Army private who volunteered for the experiment. Unlike Carroll, whose work put him in frequent contact with yellow fever, Dean was known to be nonimmune and he had been on the grounds of Columbia Barracks for nearly two months before being bitten. When Dean was diagnosed with yellow fever on September 7, it could only be attributed to the mosquito bite.[19]

On September 18, 1900, Lazear became ill with yellow fever. His case took a turn for the worse, and a week later, he succumbed to the disease.[20] According to the official account of Lazear's death, he had allowed himself to be bitten by a mosquito while visiting Las Ánimas,

Havana's yellow fever hospital. Previously, on August 16, Lazear had allowed himself to be bitten by a mosquito that had bitten a patient suffering a mild case of yellow fever ten days earlier. Reed asserted that, as he did not suffer any symptoms from that first bite, Lazear believed himself immune to yellow fever and so allowed the later bite at the hospital. This mosquito apparently infected Lazear with the yellow fever that took his life.[21] Upon hearing of Lazear's illness, Reed commented that he was disappointed that, like Carroll, Lazear could have contracted the disease from other sources at Las Ánimas, and so "2 such valuable lives have been put in jeopardy, under circumstances in which the results obtained would not be above Criticism."[22] It is, however, difficult to believe that Lazear would think himself immune after the first bite given his knowledge of the two-week extrinsic incubation period of yellow fever proven by Carter, and Reed in fact later told his wife that Lazear allowed himself to be bitten "in order to test our theory."[23]

When he heard what had happened, Reed immediately returned to Havana in early October, and using Lazear's meticulously kept notes, quickly wrote up the early mosquito experiments and the yellow fever cases of Carroll and Dean for presentation at the annual meeting of the American Public Health Association just three weeks later. On October 12, he met with Governor Wood and Major Jefferson Kean, chief surgeon of the administrative department surrounding the city of Havana, to request permission to construct a camp for conducting further human experiments of the mosquito theory, which Wood granted.[24] The next day, Reed left for the United States to present Lazear's findings.[25]

When Reed returned to Havana at the end of October he began preparing a new round of experiments. On November 20, the construction of Camp Lazear was completed, six miles from Havana, far from "any other possible source of infection."[26] Beginning that day, a series of seven nonimmune volunteers, all of whom had been quarantined to ensure that they were not already infected, were bitten by mosquitoes that had fed on yellow fever patients at least eleven days earlier. All but one developed yellow fever within days.[27]

Many of the first volunteers were recently arrived Spanish immigrants. The Yellow Fever Commission saw the Triscornia immigrant camp as a prime source for human subjects for the experiments since it had been established to keep newly arrived Spanish away from Havana where they could contract yellow fever until they found employment in the countryside. But rumors of experimentation on Spanish immigrants soon surfaced in Havana newspapers. *La Discusión* sensationally reported that scores of immigrants had been recruited to work at Camp

Lazear and then, at the end of the workday, were locked in rooms with infected mosquitoes: "If, unfortunately, this is true, this would be the most monstrous case of savagery that we have ever witnessed."[28] In actuality, only five immigrants were recruited, they had all been informed of the risk of contracting a potentially deadly case of yellow fever, and the inoculations were carefully administered using mosquitoes kept in test tubes.[29] Potential volunteers were informed, however, that it was "entirely impossible for [them] to avoid the infection during [their] stay in this island," an exaggeration that casts doubt on how well informed the consent really was.[30] Volunteers were paid one hundred dollars in gold for participating and an additional one hundred dollars if they contracted the disease.[31] If they survived yellow fever, they would also receive a certificate of immunity. Because those who could prove their immunity to yellow fever could command higher wages, this was an attractive proposition for poor Spanish immigrants.[32]

Reed soon found, however, that he was unable to recruit additional Spanish volunteers. Gorgas recalled:

> The work from being much sought had become very unpopular. For some time he was unable to find any good reason for this. The story told in Havana was that the American soldiers, who were doing the guard duty for the camp, had found an old lyme kiln in the lower part of the grounds. In this kiln they had placed a lot of bleached old bones, and here they would take the newly arrived Spaniard and darkly insinuate that these were the bones of their predecessors in Dr. Reed's camp, and that if they did not leave before they were bitten by Dr. Reed's mosquitoes, their bones would soon be bleaching in the same place. It was useless for Dr. Reed to argue and explain. This ocular evidence was too strong for any argument by word of mouth, and Dr. Reed had to give it up.[33]

From that point forward, only U.S. Army volunteers participated in the experiments and gained the two-hundred-dollar award.

Reed also designed two additional sets of experiments, and a simple frame house was built for each. The first house consisted of a single room, fourteen by twenty feet, and was tightly sealed to prevent any ventilation. On November 30, the building was filled with bedding that "had been purposefully soiled with a liberal quantity of black vomit, urine, and fecal matter" from yellow fever patients.[34] That evening, a

U.S. Army surgeon and two privates, all nonimmune, entered the house; for the next twenty nights, they slept in the contaminated beds, surrounded by the filth of yellow fever patients. None contracted yellow fever. The experiment was repeated twice more with new nonimmune volunteers in December and January, with the same results. The conclusion was clear: Fomites, materials contaminated with yellow fever, could not convey the disease.

The second house was identical in its proportions to the first one, but it was well ventilated and divided in half by a metal screen. On December 21, fifteen infected mosquitoes were released on one side of the building. One nonimmune volunteer, John J. Moran, then entered the mosquito side of the building where he remained for thirty minutes and was bitten several times. He visited the mosquito room again later that day and the next day, getting bitten both times. Meanwhile, two nonimmune volunteers began their stay at the other side of the metal screen; they slept in the house every night until January 8, 1901. On December 25, Moran fell ill with yellow fever, but the volunteers screened away from the mosquitoes never contracted the disease.

The Reed commission was confident that, together, the three sets of experiments established that yellow fever was caused only by the bite of a mosquito that had bitten a yellow fever patient more than twelve days earlier.[35] Others in the occupation government agreed. In December 1900, Gorgas wrote to Carter, by then stationed in Baltimore, that although Reed's description of Lazear's first successful cases had failed to convince him of the mosquito theory, the later experiments provided very strong evidence in its favor: "So I think if you want to be in at the killing, you had better come down this winter. I think we are about to make a historic campaign against yellow jack in Havana next summer, and such a seasoned old veteran as you ought to have part in such a climax."[36] With the confirmation by the Yellow Fever Commission of Finlay's theory as amended by Carter, the occupation government turned its attention to the mosquito.

From Theory to Practice: The Antimosquito Campaign in Havana

The work of the Yellow Fever Commission prompted a shift in the tactics the occupation government employed in its fight against yellow fever. Rather than exclusively targeting filth, the occupation focused its attention on the mosquito. Beginning in February 1901, the Sanitary Office of Havana took a new, two-pronged approach to combating yellow fever: first, it killed mosquitoes at the homes of those diagnosed with yellow fever, and second, it systematically destroyed mosquito breeding places across the city.[37]

When a case of yellow fever was identified, the patient was quarantined in one part of the home, which was screened in with a mosquito-proof wire mesh. One of Havana's two twelve-man Special Disinfection Brigades that specialized in yellow fever cases then began killing mosquitoes.[38] Every room in the house was sealed and fumigated for two to three hours with burning pyrethrum powder, which paralyzed the mosquitoes. The room was opened, and the mosquitoes on the floor were killed, swept up, and destroyed. All surrounding buildings were similarly fumigated in an effort to ensure that no infected mosquito escaped.[39] In suspect warehouses, sulfur was burned to kill any potentially infected mosquitoes, and in tobacco factories and storage facilities, tobacco smoke was used instead.[40] "The disagreeable and costly process of disinfection formerly in use has been practically done away with," wrote Governor Wood. "The means at present employed are much less destructive to property and much less annoying to the people."[41]

Destroying all of the breeding places of the mosquito in Havana was a more formidable task, and one that engendered more resistance from the city's inhabitants. In March 1901, two-thirds of the Sanitary Department's crews were reassigned from their cleaning duties to a house-to-house oiling campaign: "A little oil is placed in every receptacle containing standing water and about an ounce into every closet and sink in houses having water connections. Nearly every house in Havana has a cess-pool and these cess-pools are ideal breeding places for mosquitoes. The oil in this way runs into the cess-pool and kills the larvae."[42] About twenty thousand houses were treated in that first month.[43]

Complicating the oiling campaign was the fact that the city had no comprehensive water system: each family collected rainwater in casks or barrels for drinking purposes, and the floating oil made drawing fresh water difficult. "It was soon found that the tenants of many houses removed the oil as soon as our inspectors left the premises," Gorgas reported.[44] At the prompting of Gorgas and Wood, on May 6, 1901, the mayor of Havana ordered that all drinking water receptacles be kept oiled, covered, and fitted with a pump or stopcock so that water was drawn from the bottom; yards were to be kept drained and dry.[45] The mosquito-proofing efforts gradually expanded to also include all drains, pipes, and sewer connections.[46] These orders were widely distributed, and owners of wells and cisterns were also notified by mail to make them mosquito-proof. The city was divided into eight inspection districts, and each house was inspected once a month for compliance. Gorgas informed Wood in August 1901 that, in the early months of the campaign, the inspection crews had found it "necessary to break many barrels containing water, not made mosquito-proof according to the order. This had a very good effect, and in certain streets where water deposits used to exist in every yard, there are now none to be found."[47] Sanitary inspection crews destroyed an additional 842 rainwater barrels that were infested with mosquito larvae in August and September 1901, thereby depriving many people of their source of potable water.[48] All reports of mosquitoes were quickly addressed by the Sanitary Department.[49]

The Sanitary Department also compelled observance through legal proceedings, often bringing over a thousand cases in a single month. Gorgas explained that this

> will no doubt strike the health officer of our large cities as being very excessive. But, as I have the power of withdrawing cases, I use this measure very freely for getting the work done. If any work ordered has not been commenced on re-inspection within a week after the order is given, I start legal proceedings. This almost invariably causes the owner to commence work.[50]

By March 1902, the percentage of homes found to have larvae infestations had fallen to just 0.6 percent from nearly 100 percent a year earlier: "This would seem to indicate that by the continuous house to house inspection we can reduce the number of breeding places of the Stegomyia down to a very small number in the near future," the head of the mosquito efforts reported to Gorgas.[51]

The Sanitary Department's heavy-handed approach generated resentment among many inhabitants of Havana. Facing the confiscation of property because he had not paid a fine, one bank owner complained to Governor Wood. He stressed that he had already spent "many thousands of pesos" on "modern toilets, fosas, drainage pipes" and proceeded to denounce the "ineffective" and "perfectly useless" measures to control mosquitoes:

> the Sanitation office has invented now that one must put metallic mesh on the water reservoirs, *to exterminate the mosquito.* I do not want to offend your good judgment by ridiculing this measure, which has not even been adopted in New Orleans where the climate is analogous to ours; and it is as absurd for

the purpose it is intended for as the one where one tries to cover the sky with a finger.

Wood referred the matter to Gorgas, who directed that the legal action continue until the bank was in compliance.[52] One woman insisted that the well in her home was perfectly clean, that it harmed no one, and that the order from the sanitary authorities to install a cover and pump infringed on her rights as a property owner.[53] Others challenged the right of sanitary inspectors even to enter their homes. On the recommendation of Gorgas, Wood ordered that, when occupants denied sanitary inspectors entrance into any building, Havana police had the duty "to see that the inspector is at once admitted."[54] With the backing of the military government, the Sanitary Department would not be denied.

The mosquito-control efforts of the occupation government were soon spread to Cuba's other large cities. By July 1901, the authorities in Santiago had divided the city into inspection districts and started mosquito extermination work.[55] In Matanzas, U.S. military engineers were charged with the fight against the mosquito. Their efforts "consisted of covering with petroleum all collected water in order to stop the breeding of mosquitoes. There are seven sprayers who check all the houses in Matanzas, Pueblo Nuevo and Versalles twice a month and use up 220 gallons of petroleum monthly."[56]

Not everyone adapted quickly to the changed focus of yellow fever efforts; many government officials in Cuba and the U.S. South maintained their deeply ingrained beliefs that the disease was transmitted by fomites—infected objects—rather than mosquitoes. When informed that a yellow fever patient was being transported to the city of Matanzas for treatment, commanding officer Colonel Henry Noyes remarked, "The within case is the third case brought into the City from outlying municipalities for treatment. In each instance the cases were enroute during the period of greatest danger from infection. This practice endangers the health of this command as well as that of the City. I recommend that it be stopped." The chief surgeon of the island, Major Valerie Havard, had to reassure him that so long as the patient was kept screened from mosquitoes, transporting him into the city was perfectly safe.[57] For its part, the USMHS continued to insist on disinfecting baggage from Cuba bound for destinations south of Maryland, and the Louisiana State Board of Health reiterated that "any vessel from Cuban Ports on which undisinfected baggage is found, regardless of destination of such baggage, will be detained five full days after disinfection of such baggage, at the Mississippi Quarantine Station."[58]

Nevertheless, switching from general sanitation to mosquito eradication generated quick results in the occupation government's battle with yellow fever. The toll of yellow fever in Havana for January 1901, twenty-four cases and seven deaths, was similar to that for January 1900, when there were nineteen cases and eight deaths. With the commencement of mosquito work, the numbers began to decline: during February and March 1901, yellow fever was reported at half the rate of the previous year. "As a matter of fact," Gorgas wrote in his monthly report for March, "we have had only one case of yellow fever in Havana since the 1st of March, and since March 23rd, the city of Havana has been entirely free of the disease."[59]

March, however, marked the low point for yellow fever in Havana every year. The true test of the new campaign would come as summer approached. In April, there were only two cases of yellow fever in Havana, and both patients recovered. The health officials of the USMHS who were charged with managing the quarantine of the U.S. South against yellow fever took note: "On account of the favorable sanitary conditions of the city, the National authorities have deferred their quarantine from April 1st to May 15th, which is a great benefit to commerce and travel."[60] On May 6 and 7, four patients were diagnosed with yellow fever, but none died. The remainder of May and all of June passed with no trace of yellow fever in the city. This was truly an accomplishment; since at least 1761 no June in Havana had ever been free of yellow fever.[61]

In July, a small outbreak of yellow fever occurred in Regla, an outlying suburb of Havana, resulting in four cases and one death. The disease was traced to the small town of Santiago de las Vegas, twelve miles away on the railroad line. The Sanitary Department responded quickly, Gorgas reported: "a considerable force was put into Santiago de las Vegas, and work at once commenced in an endeavor to free the town from infection. Our efforts were made entirely in the line of destroying infected mosquitoes; in this way I hope we have been successful."[62] Other small outbreaks occurred in Havana during August and September, resulting in fourteen cases and four deaths. "This is so much better than anything that has occurred before, that we feel convinced it can only be due to the methods of disinfection adopted by order of the Military Governor; that is, the thorough destruction of infected mosquitoes in the neighborhood of the focus of infection," Gorgas wrote in September.[63] Three cases and no deaths occurred during the first week of October 1901; for the remainder of the occupation of Cuba, Havana remained free of yellow fever. Figure 7 traces the course of the disease in Havana from 1900, through the beginning of mosquito work in Febru-

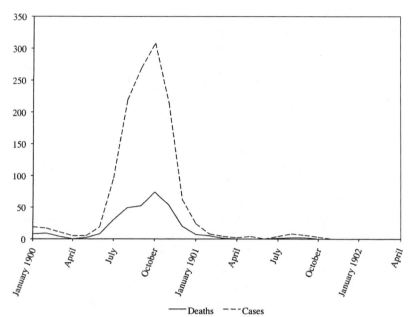

FIGURE 7 Monthly yellow fever cases and deaths in Havana, January 1900 to April 1902

ary 1901, to the end of the occupation in April 1902. The contrast of the 1901 yellow fever season with that of a year earlier is dramatic.

The measures taken to control yellow fever by destroying mosquitoes obtained similarly impressive results all over the island. At the peak of the 1901 yellow fever season, Colonel Noyes reported from Matanzas, "There has been no epidemic prevalent during the year, only a few isolated cases of yellow fever having been reported."[64] The commanding officer of the District of Santiago commented, "the sanitary condition of the towns and cities of the District is satisfactory and steadily improving. During the past twelve months there has been no epidemic traceable to unsanitary conditions. . . . There has not been a single case of yellow fever for over eight months."[65]

The rapid and complete success of the antimosquito campaign astonished even those who implemented it. "I, myself, am so entirely taken aback and surprised at the result of our mosquito work, that I hardly know what to think. It can't be chance, and yet it seems too much to expect that we could have controlled yellow fever as we have this year," Gorgas wrote in the autumn of 1901.[66] Carter, observing the progress from his new post in Baltimore, wrote Gorgas that "your success *is almost too complete to be convincing. You ought to have some [yellow fever] this year* and get rid of it in 1902 or 03."[67]

The success of the antimosquito efforts allowed the U.S. occupation government to turn some attention to lower priorities, such as tuberculosis. In March 1902, a group of Cuban doctors pleaded that tuberculosis, a "hidden plague that counts its victims by the thousand, may be easily overcome if the Government decides to make only one half of the pecuniary sacrifices so wisely used to extirpate yellow fever."[68] As shown in figure 8, tuberculosis had claimed more lives than yellow fever in Havana every year since 1890. That decade, tuberculosis claimed an average of more than 1,600 lives per year; annual yellow fever deaths averaged less than 500. In 1898, the year that U.S. authorities took control of Cuba, while 858 people died of yellow fever in Havana, 2,794 died of tuberculosis. In 1899, there were 981 reported tuberculosis deaths in Havana and only 103 yellow fever deaths. By 1901, the occupation government's antimosquito policies had virtually eliminated yellow fever; only eighteen people died from the disease that year. Conversely, there had been very little improvement in tuberculosis during the U.S. occupation; nine hundred people died of tuberculosis in 1901.[69]

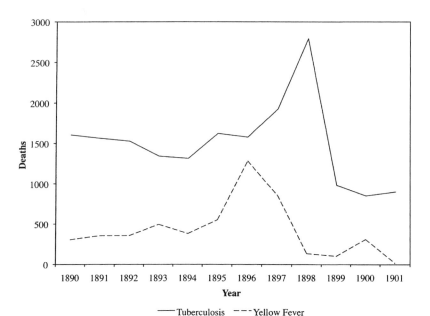

FIGURE 8 Annual tuberculosis and yellow fever deaths in Havana, 1890–1901

In response to the Cuban physicians, Gorgas wrote that, as the yellow fever wards were empty, Governor Wood "has ordered that a sanatorium for incurable cases of tuberculosis be established in the old yellow fever section of municipal hospital No. 1" in Havana.[70] Empty yellow fever beds were similarly reassigned in Santiago.[71] The previous summer twenty stations were established throughout the city of Havana in order to collect specimens for testing for tuberculosis as well as typhoid, malaria, diphtheria, glanders, and filariasis.[72] The recommendations of Cuban doctors for an educational campaign against tuberculosis were also implemented: "information as to the nature and care of this disease is being very generally spread among the people by lectures, printed matter, etc."[73] On May 9, 1902, just eleven days before the U.S. forces withdrew from Cuba, Gorgas reported that, "We have lately greatly extended our tuberculosis work, and are now in touch with almost every tuberculosis patient living in Havana. It is hoped to show a still more marked improvement in the rate from tuberculosis, if the present system can be continued."[74]

Only after Havana's endemic yellow fever was eliminated did the health officials of the occupation government address the leading cause of death on the island. The primary concern of the occupation was not the health of Cubans, but the economic stability of the U.S. South. Because tuberculosis in Cuba, unlike yellow fever, was not a threat to the United States, it was only a low priority to U.S. authorities.

: : :

After years of efforts aimed at cleaning the cities, sanitary authorities had failed to control yellow fever. It was not until the Yellow Fever Commission built on the work of Henry Carter and confirmed Carlos Finlay's theory that mosquitoes transmitted yellow fever that an effective strategy for controlling the disease could be put in place. The occupation government quickly adopted policies of destroying mosquito breeding places and preventing mosquitoes from biting yellow fever patients. The effectiveness of this new strategy was evident within months, and by the end of 1901 Cuba was virtually free of yellow fever. Contact with the island was no longer a threat to the health and economy of the U.S. South.

In his last report as Chief Sanitary Officer of the City of Havana, Gorgas wrote: "Our work down here has been a useful lesson in municipal sanitation. The same thing could be accomplished by any community anywhere else, if they were willing to spend money and labor on it. No elaborate machinery of any kind is necessary; merely men and brooms."[75] The amount of money spent on sanitation and quarantine during the occupation, however, was far from trivial: at over ten million dollars, it was the largest single item in the budget.[76] The political will necessary was also considerable. Contrasting the occupation government's success in Havana with the U.S. Public Health Service's failure to control yellow fever in Laredo, Texas, in 1903, Dr. Gregorio M. Guiteras argued that U.S. cities must declare martial law at the onset of an outbreak to be successful in using antimosquito efforts to stop the spread of the disease.[77] After his experience fighting yellow fever in the Panama Canal Zone, Gorgas came to a similar conclusion: "We thought that in one year and at all cost we might accomplish the same in Panama as in Havana, but here we did not have a military authority. The lack of cooperation on the part of the authorities caused the failure of these measures, and we had to look for other procedures in order to attain our object in dealing with yellow fever."[78]

Would the Cubans, left to their devices, expend the money and exert the political will necessary to keep yellow fever from regaining its hold on the island and again threatening the U.S. South? As leaving Cuba to the Cubans drew closer to becoming reality, many in the United States feared that the accomplishments of the occupation government in controlling yellow fever on the island would evaporate as soon as the U.S. military withdrew. Only a few months after the creation of the Cuban republic, an officer of the Florida Board of Health wrote to Gorgas with great concern:

> I hear ugly rumors of Havana Sanitary force! I hear that fully one third of the force transferred by you, has been discharged, and that already in some streets the garbage begins to look like old days before the "occupation." I mean scattered along the sidewalks. Look out for the "festive mosquito," which has been lurking the many months of waiting for the chance of her life which seems to be coming pretty soon under the state of affairs.[79]

The Floridian doctor had little cause for worry, as the U.S. government had already prepared for the event that these rumors were true: the Cuban government would maintain the sanitary standards put into place during the occupation, or the United States would invade the island again.

5

The Mosquito Threatens Independence

The only nation of the world whose independence could be threatened by a mosquito is the Republic of Cuba. **José H. Pazos, "Contribución al estudio de los mosquitos en Cuba"**

: : :

With the end of the occupation government in 1902, Cuba was at last independent, but U.S. concerns about yellow fever powerfully shaped the limits of this independence. Before relinquishing control over the island, the U.S. government demanded that the new Republic of Cuba agree to maintain the sanitary conditions necessary to prevent the spread of yellow fever to the southern United States. This demand, which has received little attention from scholars, was central to the negotiations of independence and was finally enshrined within the Platt Amendment and incorporated in the Cuban constitution.[1] The Cuban government nevertheless initially accorded low priority to yellow fever prevention, but the experiences of the first decade of the republic demonstrated that U.S. demands regarding public health could not be disregarded.

Sanitation and Independence

The U.S. occupation government, put in place following the end of Spanish rule on the island, could not remain in Cuba indefinitely. When the U.S. Congress authorized President William McKinley to intervene in the war in Cuba in 1898, it had declared,

> the people of the Island of Cuba are, and of right ought to be, free and independent[, and] the United States hereby disclaims any disposition or intention to exercise sovereignty, jurisdiction, or control over said Island, except for the pacification thereof, and asserts its determination, when that is accomplished, to leave the government and control of the Island to its people.[2]

Under this declaration, known as the Teller Resolution, the occupation government was obliged to organize a Cuban government and to relinquish control of the island.

In July 1900, President McKinley directed Governor Wood to order the formation of a constitutional convention.[3] Wood's Order 301 called for the election of thirty-one delegates to a convention "to frame and adopt a constitution for the people of Cuba, and, as part thereof, to provide for and agree with the Government of the United States upon the relations to exist between that Government and the Government of Cuba."[4]

The elections were held in September, and the new Constitutional Convention first met on November 5. Wood opened the convention by charging the delegates "first, to frame and adopt a Constitution for Cuba, and when that has been done, to formulate what, in your opinion, ought to be the relations between Cuba and the United States." The United States government, he explained, would then "take such action on its part as shall lead to a final and authoritative agreement between the people of the two countries to the promotion of their common interests."[5] Wood then left the delegates to complete their task. On February 21, 1901, the delegates signed the final copy of the new Cuban constitution, but the issue of relations with the United States had been completely omitted. Wood and Secretary of War Elihu Root, aware of the convention's lack of progress on the issue, had already taken the initiative.

On February 9, 1901, Root sent Wood a letter with his suggestions for how the relations between Cuba and the United States should be enshrined within the Cuban constitution. He listed five points. First, that the Cuban government's power to negotiate treaties would be circumscribed. Cuba would not have the power to enter treaties that "may tend to impair or interfere with the independence of Cuba, or to confer upon foreign powers any special right or privilege without the consent of the United States." Second, the Cuban government would not have the authority to borrow beyond its means. Third, the United States would have a continuing right to intervene in Cuban affairs "for the preservation of Cuban independence and the maintenance of a stable Government, adequately protecting life, property and individual liberty." Fourth, that the acts of the occupation government would be ratified. Fifth and finally, that the United States would be permitted to establish naval bases on the island.[6]

Wood agreed with these points, but believed that Root had overlooked a matter "of vital importance." The proposed conditions did not address U.S. interests in Cuban health and sanitation. After all, Wood reminded Root, "the purpose of the war was not only to assist the Cubans, but, in a general sense, to abate a nuisance," the threat of yellow fever spreading from Cuba to the U.S. South. Without a provision requiring the maintenance of good sanitation, he feared, Havana and other major Cuban cities would revert to the conditions that prevailed before the U.S. occupation of the island. Cuba would again become "a menace to our Southern seaports and the consequent interference with commerce will continue." Wood felt that the Cubans could not be trusted to continue the fight against yellow fever on their own: "As a rule, the people of the island are immune to yellow fever and, consequently, take little interest in the elaborate sanitary precautions which have been instituted under American rule." A sanitation clause was therefore essential, Wood reiterated, as the "question of control of sanitation of Cuban ports is, in my opinion, of vital importance to the United States."[7]

Root discussed Wood's concern with President McKinley and with Senators Orville Platt and John Spooner of the Senate Committee on Relations with Cuba. All agreed that sanitation was a critical issue in U.S.-Cuban relations, and, Root assured Wood, "It will not be lost sight of in the treatment of the subject here." Root noted, however, that "any sanitary control involves so great an infringement of the independence and internal government of Cuba, it is difficult to say how that can be dealt with consistently with the Teller Resolution of April 20, 1898."[8] The Teller Resolution had made Cuban independence an element of U.S. law, which barred any continuing control of the island after its pacification.[9] Because only Congress could supersede an existing law, Root pointed out, it would have to approve any sanitation clause.[10]

It is telling that sanitation raised warning flags for Root as an unlawful infringement of Cuban independence, whereas retaining a "right of intervention" for the United States in Cuban affairs did not. Root's care on the sanitation issue likely stemmed from his training as a lawyer; he had been a prominent member of the New York bar before his appointment as secretary of war. The regulation of public health was recognized as an essential element of sovereignty by nineteenth-century U.S. constitutional law.[11] Attempts to bring public health under federal control in the United States, in fact, had faced stiff opposition on the grounds that quarantine was not among the powers the sovereign states had delegated to the federal government.[12]

This argument, however, made little headway in Congress. On February 25, 1901, Senator Platt introduced the clauses as an amendment to the Army Appropriations Bill. The Platt Amendment included the original five stipulations suggested by Root, the sanitation clause added by Wood, and a provision added by Platt's committee stipulating that the status of the Isle of Pines would be settled by future treaty. Congressman Robert Wyche Davis of Florida, a Democrat, argued that the sanitation clause demanded that the Cubans'

> health laws must be made to suit us before we will remove our soldiers from their midst. And yet here at home we regard the right to make laws for the preservation of the public health as one of the reserved rights of the States. We would not think of sending an armed force into one of the States of this Union because, forsooth, its health laws or its sanitary condition might not be up to an approved standard. "That is all true," said a gentleman in discussing this matter with me the other day, "but circumstances alter cases; it is different, you know, when it comes to Cuba." Mr. Speaker, it is not different "when it comes to Cuba." Principle should control us, and not expediency. . . . "The people of the island of Cuba are, and of right ought to be, free and independent." We have said it, and let us stand to it.[13]

Charles E. Littlefield, a Republican from Maine, broke with his party to agree with Davis.[14] He pointed to the U.S. Supreme Court's recent decision in *Neely v. Henkle,* in which the Court opined that under the Teller Resolution, "exclusive control" over Cuba would be surrendered to the Cubans once they established a stable government.[15] "In section V," he observed, "in case of any change as to sanitation, [the Cubans] have no power to make it except with our consent, thus being clearly subordinate to our control in this particular. It may be conceded that if we were to exercise control over them, this subject, above all others, would be the one over which it should be exercised." Nevertheless, Littlefield concluded, "The desirability or importance of control does not demonstrate the existence of the right," and under the Teller Resolution the United States had no such right.[16]

These arguments notwithstanding, other members of Congress saw the threatened spread of disease as overriding any principle of Cuban independence or sovereignty. Congressman Richard W. Parker, a New Jersey Republican, insisted that sanitation in Cuba was "forced on us as a matter of necessity. We can no more tolerate the yellow fever in Habana than we could the protection by its government of a nest of pirates making war upon mankind." Quarantine posed too great an inconvenience in the day of high-speed transportation by steamship, Parker maintained. Continued attention to sanitation was the only solution: "Civilization itself demands that a nation or city shall not become a breeder of any plague that can be prevented."[17]

Similarly, Representative Edward L. Hamilton, a Republican from Michigan, declared that "there is nothing in this proposition restrictive of Cuban independence. The only restriction proposed is a restriction upon the spread of disease." He acknowledged that the sanitation clause "may not of right be insisted upon as a condition," but "nevertheless it ought to be acceded to by Cuba without demur as being for the common benefit of the people of Cuba and the United States."[18] Henry Gibson, the Republican congressman from Knoxville, Tennessee, asked, "Shall we have no right to guard this island . . . and see to it that the yellow fever does not use its shores as a base from which to invade our country and destroy our people?"[19]

Representative Townsend Scudder of New York made the case in favor of the sanitation clause most forcefully. "One of the chief reasons which justified this country's intervention to rescue Cuba from Spanish misrule," he reminded his colleagues, "is to be found in the fact that the deplorable sanitary condition of the island made it a dangerous nuisance. It was like having an open cesspool opposite one's front door. The thing had to be abated." Infested with yellow fever, Cuba "was a standing menace to the welfare of the American people. It involved them in periodic plagues which cost hundreds of lives, great financial loss, and brought business over a large part of the country to a standstill."[20]

Scudder pointed out that intervention and occupation had provided the United States with the opportunity, at "a very considerable expense of life and money," to eliminate this hazardous condition, and its efforts had been remarkably successful: "By the application and enforcement of modern methods of sanitation at Habana and Santiago the scourge of yellow fever has been greatly mitigated—almost stamped out."[21] The United States, the Republican legislator continued, could not afford to squander this accomplishment. Maintaining acceptable sanitary conditions in Cuba after the island became "an independent sovereignty" would be difficult, Scudder argued:

> If the Cubans ever get to control things absolutely it is not unreasonable to assume that, in the light of the past, all the sanitary improvements which have been introduced will quickly go by the board. The Cubans did not want those improvements. They did not want to be clean and healthy. They opposed the American innovations in this respect as so many assaults upon their traditional privileges and personal freedom. They preferred the old way of doing things. They liked smells; they had a fondness for dirt; they resented the deprivations to which they were subjected. If they are left quite free to do as they please they will return to the old state of things. Then the yellow-fever fiend will rage once more. This the Congress must prevent. It is one of the things that "Cuba libre" involves. It is unfortunate that Congress did not think of it from the start.[22]

Whether the clauses of the Platt Amendment would be accepted or rejected by the Cubans was of little importance, Scudder concluded, "They are acceptable to and will be accepted by the United States. They will be insisted upon by this country. The Cubans will do well also to accept them, for if they do not voluntarily agree to them they will be required involuntarily to conform to them. This Republic is done with nonsense."[23] The House approved the measure by a vote of 161 to 137.[24]

In the Senate, Hernando DeSoto Money of Mississippi, a member of the Committee on Relations with Cuba chaired by Platt, explained:

> This provision with respect to sanitation is a matter about which the people of my State are very much concerned. I have had them over and over again tell me that the Teller resolution was a mistake; that we ought to have taken possession of Cuba as a war indemnity, for the purpose of protecting the people of the Southern States from the infection of yellow fever. . . . I suppose that this clause will not be objected to by any man in the Cuban convention. They are anxious that sanitation shall be

had. Without it yellow fever will continue to infest the people of the United States, and we will be powerless, without some arrangement with the Cuban people on this point, to protect ourselves.[25]

Although the Cubans should work together with the United States to control yellow fever, they could not be trusted to follow through on their own, he claimed: "As a matter of fact, the people of Cuba are very little concerned about yellow fever. They do not have it in the country districts. In the city is it endemic, but not epidemic, and it does not every year become an epidemic." He then added, "It is because the United States has more interest in this question than Cuba has that we have asked them to allow us to participate in a plan to be devised for the protection of both countries against yellow fever. . . . This clause is the last one to which, I think, a man living in a country subject to yellow fever should object."[26] The Senate voted along party lines, approving the Platt Amendment by 43 to 20; Money, a Democrat, abstained.[27]

On March 2, 1901, the Army Appropriations Bill including the Platt Amendment was signed by President McKinley and became law. On Root's instructions, Wood informed the Cuban Constitutional Convention that the measures had been approved, that they were now the law of the United States, and that President McKinley awaited the convention's action.[28]

The prospects did not appear good. Even while the Platt Amendment was being discussed and debated in the U.S. Congress, Root had advised Wood to relay its provisions to the Cuban Constitutional Convention.[29] The convention met on February 26, 1901, to discuss them. Some members of the convention, including Diego Tamayo and Eliseo Giberga, argued that the sanitation clause dealt with a legitimate international concern, served a humanitarian interest, and would benefit both nations. Manuel Sanguily and Juan Gualberto Gómez insisted, however, that the clause questioned the competency of the new Cuban government and so did not even merit discussion, far less inclusion in the constitution. Even modified to encompass only future agreements between Cuba and the United States, the sanitation clause was soundly rejected by the delegates.[30]

The convention met again on March 7 to formulate a response to the by-then-enacted Platt Amendment. Some members of the convention resisted doing anything, arguing that they did not have the power to make agreements with the United States. That power, they felt, could only be properly exercised by the Cuban government to be established under the new constitution. Sanguily went as far as to call for the convention to dissolve itself immediately. Ultimately, however, they created a committee entrusted with the task of formulating a response to the U.S. government regarding the amendment.[31]

The convention reconvened on April 1 and proceeded to discuss the response to the Platt Amendment that had been proposed by the committee and the seven others offered by members of the convention. The scope of debate was marked at one end by Gómez, whose proposal was the most confrontational, and at the other by Giberga, whose response was considered the most favorable toward the Platt Amendment. Despite their differences, both delegates agreed that sanitation was a matter that the United States would have to negotiate with the new Cuban government. Gómez proposed that the government established by the new constitution

> will agree with the United States on measures to facilitate exchange between both countries, adopting, in the first instance, those resolutions of international and private hygiene that will lead to the extinction of importable diseases, as well as so many as will contribute to the development of mercantile and social relations.[32]

Giberga argued that although the sanitation clause addressed a humanitarian need and would be useful to both countries, the sanitary plans already enacted by the occupation government were completely unknown and could not be approved until after the new Cuban government had had the opportunity to examine them. They could then, like any additional plans, be the subject of a formal agreement between Cuba and the United States.[33] Apparently unaware of the importance of the sanitation issue to the U.S. government, both Gómez and Giberga expressed the belief that these formulations would be acceptable to the United States.

The convention was divided among the eight proposals, and none received majority support. Part of the reason why the delegates could not agree on an appropriate response, it seemed, was that they could not agree on what exactly the provisions of the amendment meant. Deadlocked by these issues of interpretation, the delegates agreed to send a commission of five members to Washington to get an explanation of the Platt Amendment and to negotiate terms agreeable to both sides.[34]

Domingo Méndez Capote, Rafael Portuondo, Pedro Betancourt, Diego Tamayo, and Pedro González Llorente arrived in Washington on

April 24. The following day President McKinley introduced them to Root, whom he authorized to speak officially in his name. On April 26 the delegates met again with Root to discuss questions about U.S. intervention in Cuba as permitted by the amendment. Root assured the delegates that intervention was a guarantee of U.S. protection of Cuban independence and not, as many had indicated and feared, an act of imperialism over the island. In this context the issue of sanitation was raised by the Cuban delegation. Betancourt and Tamayo wanted clarification as to what was meant by sanitation plans already established. The people of the island, they argued, could not reasonably be expected to agree to carry out a policy before learning what exactly it entailed. According to the delegates, Root responded by stating that "there were currently no established plans and that the clause referred to those [plans] that could be reached by mutual agreement between the U.S. and Cuban governments."[35] Satisfied with Root's explanations, the delegates returned to Cuba to convince their fellow members of the convention to pass the Platt Amendment.

To gain majority support, an annotated version of the Platt Amendment, including what the Cubans understood to be Root's explanations and interpretations of each clause, was proposed on May 25. About the sanitation clause, it said, "That the fifth clause refers to the measures and plans that will be mutually agreed upon by the Government of the Republic of Cuba and that of the United States."[36] It was sent to Wood and the press on May 26.[37]

Wood, concerned by the interpretations incorporated into this proposal, immediately translated the document and sent it to Root by telegram just after midnight.[38] On May 27 the delegates agreed they would vote on the proposal the following day.

Root was not pleased with the proposed appendix to the Cuban constitution. He wrote Wood on May 28, "It is in many respects very objectionable. In the first place, the acceptance of the Platt amendment is surrounded by such a cloud of words, by way of recitals and explanations, that it is difficult to tell what the real meaning is." He found the explanation of the sanitation clause, in particular, to be troubling:

> I think the explanations annexed to the acceptance of the amendment do, in substance, change the amendment. This is notably so in regard to the fifth clause, concerning sanitary measures, and the sixth clause, regarding naval bases. The fifth clause of the statute refers to sanitary plans already devised. They cannot be

> omitted. . . . I do not think that the passage of the proposed ap-
> pendix to the constitution, as transmitted to me by you, would
> be such an acceptance of the Platt amendment as to authorize
> the President's withdrawing the army from Cuba.[39]

Root's objections, however, arrived too late. By a vote of fifteen to fourteen, the Constitutional Convention approved their annotated version of the Platt Amendment that same day.[40] Outraged by this turn of events, Root met with President McKinley and Senators Platt and Spooner to discuss how to respond.[41] McKinley then called a cabinet meeting. The cabinet concluded that the Cubans' treatment of the sanitation issue, along with those regarding naval bases and intervention, was unacceptable. Therefore, the U.S. government decided to reject the passing of an annotated amendment by the convention. The president directed Root to deliver the objection to the Cubans, and that afternoon Root wrote a carefully drafted letter to Wood detailing the U.S. objections to the amendment as passed.[42] He elaborated on the defects of the sanitation clause as accepted by the Cubans:

> The act of Congress calls for a provision requiring the govern-
> ment of Cuba to execute, and so far as possible extend, the plans
> already devised or other plans to be mutually agreed upon, for
> the sanitation of the cities of the island. The explanation de-
> clares that this clause refers only to plans to be mutually agreed
> upon between the government of Cuba and that of the United
> States, thus excluding from the provision all existing plans for
> sanitation and leaving no obligation whatever in regard to sani-
> tation unless Cuba chooses to agree to it hereafter. Several such
> plans now exist; some of them are in actual course of execution;
> public proposals by contractors for the execution of the com-
> pleted plans for the sanitation of Havana have recently been
> received and are under consideration. The act of Congress calls
> for a provision that all of these plans shall be executed unless
> others are substituted in their places by agreement. The provi-
> sion as accepted with the explanation would carry no obligation
> to execute them in any event.[43]

The *New York Times* identified the root of the concern for the Cuban refusal to agree to continue the existing sanitary measures. After reviewing the success of the antimosquito campaign in ridding Havana of yellow fever, the paper reminded its readers that "all that has been done is a benefaction to ourselves, as well as to the Cubans, since it decreases the danger of infection for our Southern coast ports." By limiting the sanitation clause, the convention put all this at risk: "If any argument were needed to show the folly of the Cuban Constitutional Convention in seeking to annul the sanitary clause of the Platt resolutions, the wonderful regeneration of Havana under Major Gorgas's masterly administration furnishes an all-sufficient one."[44]

The United States responded to the Cuban action with an ultimatum, and Wood formally transmitted the U.S. position on June 8. He reiterated Root's insistence that the Platt Amendment was U.S. law and that, therefore, the president had no power to change or modify it. Unless the Cubans accepted its provisions exactly as they appeared, President McKinley was not authorized to withdraw the U.S. forces from the island.[45] On June 12, the Cuban Constitutional Convention voted on the amendment without modification and passed it by a vote of sixteen to ten.[46]

Why did members of the convention pass the Platt Amendment with annotations that made it unacceptable to the United States? There are three possible explanations. The first maintains that the Cubans were trying to modify the Platt Amendment's terms so as to ameliorate the extent of its infringements of Cuban sovereignty. By making the sanitation clause apply only to future agreements between Cuba and the United States, the convention's version avoided binding the new Cuban government to continue the existing measures combating yellow fever. This was the view of many contemporary observers in the United States. The *New York Times* opined that the convention delegates took "that view of the amendment that best suit[ed] their personal convenience and political plans," and simply lied about their conversations with Root to justify their actions.[47] Indeed, some observers in the United States had long suspected that the Cubans were attempting to avoid making any commitments whatsoever.[48]

A second view holds that the members of the convention were simply trying to put down the meaning of the terms of the agreement as they understood them from their conversations with Root and Wood. According to this view, the U.S. officials had attempted to sugarcoat the terms of the amendment to induce the Cubans to pass it and then were caught in their lies when the Cubans put their words to paper. Diego Tamayo and Méndez Capote were reportedly disappointed with the U.S. rejection; they were sure that what was passed by the convention would be acceptable to the U.S. government because they had merely incorporated the explanations offered by Wood and Root.[49] The *New*

York Evening Post reported that the Cuban convention had "left Secretary Root looking uncommonly foolish" as "all his private assurances to the delegates who went to Washington, all his labored explanations of the intent of the Platt Amendment, they have incorporated in the majority report and propose to make a part of the binding agreement between Cuba and the United States!"[50] For his part, Root vehemently denied the explanations attributed to him by the Cubans.[51]

While possible, it is unlikely that the Cuban delegates used their explanations of the amendment as an attempt to sneak their absolute independence by the U.S. government. It is also unlikely that Root would tell the delegates that their interpretations of the amendment were acceptable. Instead, the best explanation is that the Cuban and U.S. officials hurled denunciations and pointed fingers at each other because neither side could understand the other's position on the issue. The Cubans failed to recognize the importance of the sanitation clause to the United States. The annotation to the sanitation clause reflected a misunderstanding that arose from the Cubans' lack of appreciation of the importance of the sanitation issue to the United States. For the Cubans, yellow fever was a disease that affected mostly foreigners and was therefore hardly a pressing national priority. To the United States, on the other hand, yellow fever was a critical concern. The threat of yellow fever was an important motivation for the U.S. entry into the war against Spain, the occupation government had gone to great lengths to eradicate the disease, and the U.S. government was unwilling to risk losing the consequent benefits to the U.S. economy to the indifference of a Cuban government.

On May 20, 1902, Wood delivered his final message to the president and congress of the new Republic of Cuba. He announced the end of the occupation and the transfer of government and control of the island to the Cuban people. As his final words as military governor of the island, Wood reminded the Cubans that they were bound to maintain the already established plans for the sanitation of the island in accordance with the Platt Amendment and the new Cuban constitution.[52] Cuban President Tomás Estrada Palma accepted the transfer and acknowledged his government's responsibility to uphold the standards of sanitation established by the military government.[53]

Early Tensions

It did not take long, however, for matters of sanitation to become a source of tension between the two countries. Only days after the withdrawal of U.S. forces from the island, the new U.S. minister to Cuba, Herbert G. Squiers, expressed his concern for the Cuban government's commitment to sanitation. In his first address to the Cuban legislature, Estrada Palma said that although the current state of sanitation was good, steps to ensure these favorable conditions were made permanent were still needed. "The promises made to guarantee the absolute eradication of yellow fever, as an indicator of an exceptionally sanitary condition," Estrada Palma noted, "could be undertaken because we are talking about a problem of such magnitude that it is not only related to our internal social order but it also demands serious attention on the international front."[54] Squiers was not satisfied. He complained to John Hay, the secretary of state, "Regarding the matter of sanitation, the matter seems to be passed over very lightly and not given that importance which the necessity certainly demands."[55]

Part of Squiers's disappointment may have resulted from misunderstanding Estrada Palma's speech. In the translation Squiers sent to Hay the sentence quoted above read, "The means taken for procuring the entire disappearance of yellow fever as the exponent of an exceptional sanitary condition, may perhaps be successful, inasmuch as they treat of a programme of such magnitude as not only to relate to the internal welfare, but to claim serious consideration as regards the international wellbeing."[56] In contrast to Estrada Palma's powerful reaffirmation of the importance of fulfilling Cuba's commitment to sanitation, Squiers understood a jumbled comment on the measures previously adopted.

Whatever the source of Squiers's misgivings, concern about a deteriorating sanitary situation was also shared by other U.S. officials. Gorgas, who had remained in Havana, complained that, "sanitation is not being kept at all up to our standards." He did, however, trust the new chief sanitary officer of Havana, Carlos J. Finlay, to maintain the antimosquito work, "so that I believe that Havana will keep free of yellow fever, even if the general sanitation becomes pretty bad."[57]

Indeed, in November 1902, Estrada Palma reported to the Cuban congress that, "the greatest vigilance is carefully exercised by the sanitary officers to avoid the reappearance of yellow fever."[58] The U.S. Marine Hospital Service (USMHS) officials stationed around the island agreed. They applauded "the very excellent quarantine methods adopted by the quarantine authorities of Cuba."[59] In Matanzas, the USMHS quarantine officer reported, "The good sanitary work in the city continues under the direction of its efficient health officer, Dr. Alberto Schweyer. The streets are kept clean, garbage is collected daily, inspection of houses made every day. . . . No accumulation of filth is tolerated anywhere."[60]

The sanitary condition of Nuevitas "is and has been excellent through-out the year."[61] In Santiago de Cuba, it was reported that, "taken as a whole, the health of the city has been good." The creation of a mosquito brigade, "whose business is to make an inspection of the houses and streets and drain or put crude petroleum wherever they deem it neces-sary in order to kill the larvae of mosquitoes," was especially lauded: "This is a permanent organization, with a sufficient appropriation to do the work well."[62] The lack of a similar effort in Cienfuegos, where mosquitoes "abound in great numbers," was worrisome, but the city was free of yellow fever, "and with a continuance of the present strict quarantine maintained against infected ports there is not likely to be any introduced through this port."[63]

The Cuban government's initial concern for sanitation, however, soon gave way to neglect. Congressional appropriations for sanitation, generous in the first year of the republic, disappeared in its second year. The results were quickly evident. In Matanzas, the USMHS officer re-ported that the lack of funding caused two-thirds of the city's sanitation force to be discharged, "including the mosquito brigades, the force in charge of the daily irrigation of the streets, and that devoted to the house-to-house inspection. The outcome of all of this can readily be foreseen if the existing conditions are not corrected in time."[64] Santiago de Cuba suffered a similar fate. In the absence of the appropriation, "the city has had a hard struggle to clean the streets, remove the garbage, and attend to other sanitary matters." The mosquito brigade "was very short lived," reported the USMHS officer: "Early in August, 1903, it was abolished for lack of funds."[65] In Cienfuegos, "the sanitary condition of the city at present is very bad in many sections" resulting in a "great increase of sickness." Moreover, "mosquitoes of all varieties abound in great numbers in all parts of the city, and no effort has been made in looking to their destruction."[66]

The deterioration of the island's sanitary condition quickly became a matter of diplomatic concern. In October 1904, the U.S. consuls of both Matanzas and Santiago de Cuba informed their superiors in the U.S. em-bassy in Havana that sanitary conditions had become intolerable. "The prevailing opinion here," William W. Hadley wrote from Matanzas, "is that a word from you to the proper authorities at Habana, pointing out the urgent need of immediate legislation to remedy the evils of this city, would have more weight and accomplish more good than the combined efforts of the local authorities."[67] In Santiago de Cuba, C. E. Little com-plained, "It is the same old story—lots of promises, but no money—so nothing can be done."[68] Their protests were immediately forwarded to Secretary of State John Hay.

That the U.S. government would take action was assured on November 11 when word reached Washington that there was yellow fever in Santiago de Cuba. Secretary of the Treasury L. M. Shaw forwarded this information to Hay and urged the State Department to bring the matter "promptly to the attention of the sanitary authorities of Cuba in order that quarantine measures, vexatious and expensive, might not be required to be enforced by the United States authorities."[69] Hay then directed Squiers, "You will point out to the Cuban Government in unmistakable terms that, unless some efficient system of ensuring good sanitary conditions for the cities of Matanzas and Santiago shall be carried out before the beginning of the active quarantine season of the coming year, it may and will probably become necessary for this Government to declare quarantine against Cuban ports."[70]

The next day, the situation grew worse. Another case of yellow fever was found in Santiago de Cuba and the U.S. consul to the city quickly informed his superiors.[71] On November 28 Squiers met with President Estrada Palma, who assured the minister that a thorough investigation of the situation in Santiago de Cuba would be undertaken and the money needed for sanitation would be disbursed.[72] But Santiago de Cuba was not the only city with problems. The U.S. consul in Cárdenas reported abundant "breeding places for myriads of mosquitoes with which the town is cursed, and of which, I am told, it is never without." Although there was not yet any sign of yellow fever, "once attacked yellow fever would take a strong hold"; he concluded: "Radical measures should be taken immediately."[73]

The situation was drawing the attention of other foreign observers as well. Raphaël Blanchard, French specialist in tropical medicine, noted the gradual increase of yellow fever cases in Cuba and reached a pointed conclusion. In his encompassing work on mosquitoes, their relationship to disease, and the public health measures used to eradicate them, he remarked,

> It is dreadful for the young Cuban republic, that if such a menacing situation does not stop promptly, the United States will see in it the opportunity to apply a certain clause from the treaty through which it consecrated Cuban independence, the clause which permits them to intervene militarily in case of political—or sanitary—disorder. It would be truly interesting

and excessive if Cuba someday loses its independence because
of the Stegomyia![74]

The choice facing the Cuban government was stark, according to
Blanchard: clean up immediately or the United States would intervene
and do the cleaning.

Cubans recognized the threat. U.S. concerns regarding sanitation in
Cuba made the front page of the Havana newspaper *La Lucha*. Insisting
that the health conditions on the island were good, Antonio San Miguel,
editor of the paper, saw an ulterior motive in U.S. accusations of declining conditions. "Is their object," he asked, "to put into practice the
Platt Amendment, inciting an intervention on sanitary grounds?"[75] The
public health of the island, he insisted, could not be neglected: "Cuba
needs to be alert and take care not to provide the smallest pretext for the
Washington administration to believe, for any reason, that the moment
has come for a second intervention."[76]

Heeding these warnings, and under pressure from the U.S. government, the Cuban congress appropriated $326,000 for the sanita-
tion of the island's cities.[77] With renewed funding, the sanitation of
Cuban cities improved.[78] The episode, however, led U.S. government
officials to conclude that relying on annual appropriations for sanitation was not enough assurance that Cuba would remain free of yellow
fever.

They began focusing on the permanent sanitary improvements in the
form of public works that had been planned by Leonard Wood in the
last year of the U.S. occupation. Three large projects had been planned:
sewers and paving of streets in Havana, sewers for Santiago de Cuba,
and waterworks for Santiago de Cuba.[79] In the absence of sewers, people relied on cesspools for the disposal of waste; these cesspools had
to be oiled regularly if they were not to become breeding grounds for
the mosquitoes that carried yellow fever. Similarly, without waterworks,
people relied on rain barrels and cisterns that local sanitation officials
also had to carefully oil and inspect for proper screen covers. Although
contracts for these projects were signed during the occupation, the work
was to commence only after the new Cuban government provided the
necessary funds.

On March 10, 1905, Secretary of State Hay wrote a detailed letter to
Squiers outlining the U.S. argument for immediate action by the Cuban
government. The public works were required by the Platt Amendment,
he explained:

The ports and commerce of the United States have heretofore
suffered immense losses through the prevalence of yellow fever
in Cuba and the importation of the same into the United States
from such sources of infection. The result has been that certain
portions of the South, at different times, have been completely
cut off by quarantine and other regulations from all social and
commercial intercourse with the other sections, with a resulting
great loss and damage to the people of the United States. In con-
sequence, the United States Government, in granting liberty to
Cuba, provided, by the covenants contained in the Platt amendment, that the evil arising from the unsanitary conditions of the
ports of the island should be remedied as soon as possible by
proper sanitary works.[80]

He directed Squiers "to bring this matter to the attention of the Government of Republic of Cuba and to urge upon it the great interest
which the United States Government has in the sanitation of the cities
of the island of Cuba."[81] Repeated demands over the next year were
met with little more than assurances by the Cuban government that the
work would be undertaken when municipal finances allowed.[82] President Estrada Palma acknowledged Cuba's obligation to undertake the
sanitation projects, but representatives from the other provinces were
reluctant to pay for improvements in Havana.[83]

The events of the autumn of 1905 underscored the importance of
making permanent sanitary improvements. On October 17 the first case
of yellow fever was diagnosed in Havana; in the span of three months,
seventy-six cases of the disease were identified. Before the epidemic
was brought under control in the city the next February, twenty-six
people had died.[84] Exacerbating the problem, Spanish immigrants passing through Havana carried the disease to Matanzas, where there were
eight confirmed cases of yellow fever and four deaths.[85] Cubans blamed
the outbreak on the failure of sanitary authorities in New Orleans to
publicize the presence of yellow fever in that city. They pointed to their
eventual success in controlling the disease as evidence that the current
sanitary measures were adequate and that the costly permanent improvements demanded by the United States were unnecessary.[86]

The continuing reticence of the Cuban government to begin the
sewer and waterworks projects infuriated newly appointed Secretary
of State Elihu Root. The Cuban response was "very unsatisfactory, in
that it gives little promise or assurance of an early compliance with the

treaty engagements. This Government thinks the time has come when there should be action. You will so inform the Cuban Government," he instructed the U.S. legation in Havana.[87] Despite Root's harsh words, the Cuban government maintained its position. Secretary of State and Justice Juan F. O'Farrill replied that Havana could not afford a loan in the amount needed to cover the sewerage contract. They argued that the present sanitary measures kept Cuba in the best possible public health and that the Cuban Congress would soon consider a bill providing the necessary funds.[88]

The yellow fever infection continued to smolder in the interior of the island. The Cuban government undertook "special sanitary and disinfecting work . . . to stamp out the yellow fever contagion" in the towns of Bolondrón, Unión de Reyes, and Alacranes, while the U.S. government kept a close eye on what was being done.[89] The Cuban efforts, however, were limited by the political unrest that followed the reelection of Estrada Palma, which had been marred by widespread fraud and other irregularities.[90]

On September 29, 1906, after two weeks of fruitless negotiations and the resignation of Estrada Palma, U.S. envoy William H. Taft announced that the United States had intervened and assumed control over the Cuban government.[91] The disorder had already allowed yellow fever to spread. By the time of Taft's announcement, the disease was again epidemic in Havana.[92]

Learning a Colonial Responsibility

Besides resolving the political unrest, the top priority of the U.S. provisional governor of Cuba, Charles E. Magoon, was the sanitation of the island.[93] Although sanitary measures in Havana quickly quelled the epidemic in the city, yellow fever proved difficult to eradicate elsewhere.[94] As U.S. adviser to the Cuban Sanitary Department Jefferson R. Kean observed, "Conquered in the centres of population, the disease has adopted revolutionary tactics and taken to the woods, and this extension to the small towns, villages and plantations brings up new and troublesome problems."[95] Yellow fever had gained a firm foothold in Matanzas in 1906 and subsequently "spread eastward until foci had been reported in every province of the Republic, except Pinar del Río."[96]

The persistent survival of yellow fever in the interior of the island underscored the deficiencies of the existing sanitary organization. Under the direct control of the national government, the sanitation of Havana had maintained acceptable standards since the beginning of the republic. The sanitation of the rest of the island, however, was left to the control of municipal authorities that did not have the same resources to expend on sanitation as the capital city did. Moreover, political considerations often hampered the enforcement of sanitary regulations at the municipal level:

> Upon trial it was found that the plan of having the local sanitary officers appointed by and subject to removal by the municipal authorities resulted in the sanitary services being improperly performed or entirely omitted. . . . The officer attempting to enforce the law usually becomes involved in difficulty with the offender and complaints to higher authority, which frequently result in reproofs, restraints and, sometimes, dismissal. Not infrequently the offender is a municipal official and the sanitary officers are unwilling to bring him to account for fear of losing their places.[97]

The spread of yellow fever to the small towns of the interior made these conditions intolerable to the U.S. authorities.

In 1907, for the first time since the end of the first U.S. occupation of Cuba, quarantine was imposed against ships leaving all ports of the island for U.S. ports south of the southern border of Maryland.[98] Beginning May 28, only immune passengers and those nonimmune persons who had remained under USMHS observation for five days before traveling were permitted to board, and the ships, cargo, and baggage were fumigated when departing from Cuba for the U.S. South.[99] This quarantine was extended beyond the end of the usual quarantine season, October 31, because of the continued presence of yellow fever on the island: "The number of cases is small, to be sure, but it is not the number of cases but their continued occurrence and the apparent impossibility of eradicating the infection, that excites alarm from a quarantine point of view in the minds of the officers of the Public Health Marine Hospital Service," stressed the U.S. secretary of the treasury.[100] Magoon was sensitive to Cuban complaints about the severity of the quarantine. He complained to Secretary of War Taft:

> The continuance of the quarantine works great injury to all interests in the island and occasions great embarrassment to the Provisional Administration. The general public here are aware that never before even in times when yellow fever was epidemic in Havana has the quarantine been maintained at this season of

the year. . . . Sanitation in Cuba is relatively of greater importance
and stands on a different basis than in the United States.[101]

The quarantine was finally lifted on December 16.

During the same year, the U.S. Provisional Government of Cuba had
been making changes in the administration of sanitation in order to
control and combat the spread of yellow fever. On August 26, 1907, it
abolished the municipal boards of health and transferred control over
sanitation to the national government and the National Board of Sanitation was established September 2.[102] Under the new system, the local
sanitary officer in each municipality reported directly to, and could rely
on the resources of, the chief sanitary officer of Cuba who, since the
beginning of the republic, had been Carlos J. Finlay. The nationalization
of sanitation allowed the extension of the techniques used to combat
yellow fever in Havana to the rest of the island. By the end of 1907, the
U.S. authorities planned

> a vigorous mosquito war for the next six months in every city,
> town, village and plantation in which the disease has appeared
> this year. . . . The smaller towns will be taught the technical
> detail of mosquito work by frequent visits of inspection, and
> this will be aided by the more efficient conduct of the sanitary
> services of street-cleaning, removal of garbage etc., which are to
> be expected under the new organization.[103]

These efforts were successful throughout most of the island. Yellow fever was eradicated in the city of Cienfuegos in January 1908 and the
province of Santa Clara in February. Only in Santiago did the infection
persist: one case was diagnosed each month from January to June.[104]

Despite the undeniable progress against yellow fever in Cuba, fears
that the disease would again spread to the U.S. South prompted action
in the United States. On March 4, the USMHS issued a department cir-
cular announcing that quarantine would be imposed against all Cuban
ports on April 1 "on account of the presence of yellow fever and uneasi-
ness as to the prevalence of the disease in various parts of the island."[105]
The provisional government protested such a harsh quarantine against
the entire island. Kean argued that there was no reason for a quarantine
against Cuba: none of the Cuban ports were then infected with yellow
fever, and, in fact, "in Havana the warfare against stegomyia mosquitoes has been so successful that it is impossible to infect it."[106] If any
quarantine was necessary, Magoon argued, it should exclude Havana

and its suburbs.[107] After these protests, the beginning of the quarantine was delayed until April 6; the city of Havana and its suburbs were exempted.[108]

Over most of the island, the efforts of the newly reorganized Board of Sanitation appeared to be a complete success. Not a single case of yellow fever occurred in five of the six Cuban provinces during the summer of 1908.[109] In Santiago, however, an outbreak of the disease began at the end of June; twenty cases occurred before August 15.[110] Despite the absence of yellow fever, the quarantine was maintained against the provinces of Pinar del Río, Havana, Matanzas, and the Isle of Pines until the beginning of August, and against the provinces of Santa Clara and Camagüey until September 10.[111] A last case of yellow fever occurred in the province of Oriente in the final week of August. When a single case was reported in the city of Havana in mid September, the USMHS reimposed quarantine against the entire island. The National Board of Sanitation was outraged. On September 17, the day after the quarantine was announced, the board passed a resolution of protest to the U.S. authorities arguing that the quarantine was an unjustified overreaction. In response to the protest, the quarantine was lifted everywhere except Santiago, where the quarantine was in effect until October 20.[112]

Yellow fever was surely a problem in 1908, but the provisional government had succeeded in eradicating the disease in Cuba. "Since this last date," Chief Sanitary Officer Finlay wrote in reference to the early September case in Havana, "in view of the radical measures that have been adopted and the care in which all non-immunes with fever are watched, there is every reason to believe that the yellow fever infection has now been stamped out."[113] The measures had indeed been radical. Over $1.1 million were spent in combating yellow fever during the occupation.[114] An additional $2.2 million were spent on general sanitation; "It is therefore a very conservative statement to say that the Provisional Government has spent more than one-tenth of the national income on sanitation," Magoon wrote.[115] In contrast to the three annual house inspections that Chief Sanitary Officer Gorgas had instituted in Havana during the first U.S. occupation of the island, an average of more than eighteen inspections per house were conducted in the city during 1908.[116] Antimosquito measures, once limited to the major cities of the island, were extended to towns and villages throughout the countryside.[117] Moreover, the provisional government built public works across Cuba to permanently reduce the threat of yellow fever. The sewering of Havana, required by the Platt Amendment, was finally begun during the summer of 1908; Magoon observed,

> With the completion of the sewer system and the abolition of
> the cesspools which now exist in connection with almost every
> house, the prevention of mosquitoes breeding will be greatly
> facilitated, and it is believed that it will be easy to keep the ste-
> gomyia mosquitoes permanently below the yellow fever limit—
> that is, below the limit of the number at which the spread of
> yellow fever becomes practicable.[118]

The Public Works Department also built a new sewer and waterworks
in Cienfuegos; Camagüey, Santiago de Cuba, and numerous towns received new supplies of water, reducing the use of rain barrels where
mosquitoes could breed.[119] These infrastructural improvements, Magoon reminded the Cubans in his final message as provisional governor,
had to be completed and maintained for Cuba to remain in compliance
with its obligations under the Platt Amendment.[120]

                                  : : :

By the end of January 1909, the provisional government had resolved
not only the political turmoil in Cuba, but also what was perceived in
Washington as the island's public health problems. In a span of three
years, it eradicated yellow fever and eliminated the conditions that allowed the disease a foothold less than a day's journey from the ports
of the southern United States. The provisional government had also
achieved a more profound transformation, one in the minds of Cubans.
Unlike the Cuban Congress of 1903, which had focused on issues of
immediate importance to a young Cuban republic while neglecting sanitation, the Cuban administration taking office with the departure of
Magoon in 1909 had learned that it must always consider the public
health concerns of the United States.

In the first year of the provisional government, the single-minded efforts to eradicate yellow fever could be publicly criticized:

> It is ridiculous that whole orders are being given continually to
> prevent the propagation of the mosquito; while it is required
> that covers be placed on the deposits of water *ad hoc;* while the
> employees of the Sanitary Department walk up and down put-
> ting petroleum in the gutters and drains, and even in the scant
> deposits of water that the resident may get in order that he shall
> not die of thirst; that focus of infection called the slaughter-

house goes on threatening death to all those that of necessity
must remain in it for any time.[121]

By 1909, however, Cubans had learned that sanitation against yellow
fever was a paramount concern to the United States and therefore must
be the paramount sanitary concern of Cuba. Under the Platt Amendment, the yellow-fever mosquito could indeed threaten the independence of Cuba. Cuban public health officials knew that "any Cuban
indifferent to the extinction of the mosquito could be judged a traitor
to his country."[122] Although yellow fever did not invade Cuba or the
United States again, its past and potential future threat continued to
influence the relationship between Cuba and its "nervous neighbors to
the north."[123]

6 The Limits of Domination

As to the debt we owe the United States for enabling us to bring about these [public health] results, we can only repay it by doing precisely what you are not willing to concede that we are doing—maintaining the standard. I hope that you may be able to establish these standards in many of your states.

Juan Guiteras, "Health Conditions in Cuba"

The talented men of the Commission demonstrated brilliantly the truth of the ideas of Finlay. They did nothing more. **Emilio Roig de Leuchsenring,** **"Reiteradamente la obra de Finlay es negada o desconocida en los Estados Unidos"**

: : :

By the end of its second military occupation of Cuba in January 1909, the United States had succeeded in eliminating a longstanding threat to the health and economy of its southern states: yellow fever in Havana. The U.S. government had demonstrated to the Cuban government, public health officials, and doctors that failing to keep the island absolutely free of yellow fever would result in economically devastating quarantine measures—whether justified by circumstances or not—and, in all likelihood, reoccupation by U.S. military forces. Faced with unremitting pressure from an overwhelming foreign power, the Cubans remained on guard against a disease that had only rarely afflicted their fellow citizens so as to protect those who lived on the opposite shore of the Gulf of Mexico.

Cubans did not, however, accept that this state of affairs was natural and appropriate. Public health officials vehemently denied the endless claims of the U.S. press that Cubans were inherently dirty, unconcerned with sanitation, and covering up continuing yellow fever infestations. Sanitarians refused to overlook the failure of their counterparts in the southern United States to even attempt to undertake the measures that would ensure that yellow fever could never affect that region. They also rejected U.S. portrayals of the breakthrough in the fight against yellow fever as an accomplishment of U.S. scientists alone and insisted on the recognition of the fundamental contribution of their countryman, Carlos J. Finlay. In short, Cubans refused to accept that U.S. control over the public health policy of their country was legitimate. The United States had achieved domination over the island, but not hegemony.

Imperialism and Hegemony

The theory of hegemony elaborated by Antonio Gramsci contends that rulers can only legitimate their power by providing benefits to those they rule in return for loyalty. When rulers supply sufficient benefits to secure the belief among the ruled that no alternative exists that could improve their situation, the existing relations of power are legitimated: domination is stable, therefore, when the dominated internalize and accept it. To achieve this state of hegemony, rulers must incorporate the aims and interests of the ruled with their own desires and interests or must convince them that what is done is in their own interests. Domination may be achieved through sheer force alone, but it can only be legitimated through a complex negotiation in which rulers convince, cajole, and make concessions to the ruled.[1]

The concept of hegemony, formulated in terms of the workings of class domination, has proven useful to the understanding of domination on the scale of nations. Colonialism similarly depends on the negotiation of power relations in a variety of daily interactions for the provision of legitimization. The successful imperialist power, like any ruler, cannot rely primarily on the forceful physical subordination of those it dominates to maintain its superior position. Rather, the imperialist must convince its colonial subjects that it is providing benefits to them that they cannot attain in any other way. Frantz Fanon, writing on French colonialism in Algeria, noted, "colonization, having been built on military conquest and the police system, sought a justification for its existence and the legitimization of its persistence in its works."[2] Successful control of a colonized people hinges on the generation of a deeply ingrained perception of dependence. As Octave Mannoni has expressed, the colonial hierarchy is itself held together by pervasive "bonds of dependence" that are embedded by the experience of colonialism.[3] Colonialism is, therefore, only validated through the acceptance by the colonized of his relationship of dependence upon the imperialist power. In the words of Albert Memmi, "Nothing legitimizes better the privilege of the colonizer than his work, nothing justifies better the ruin of the colonized than his inactivity."[4] The informal imperialism of the United States, no less than the overt colonialism of the European powers, relied upon the acceptance of the people it dominated for its legitimacy.[5]

Many Cubans saw the risk of U.S. hegemony early in the first occupation. In 1900, Cuban physician Manuel Delfín decried the effect of the public health efforts of the occupation on his fellow citizens:

> The U.S. intervention government has an extraordinary absorbing spirit; it wants to manipulate everything and presents our incompetence as pretext; and we entertain ourselves by discrediting each other; to such an extent that there is no Cuban left with a healthy bone; even if they paid us we could not have done a more perfect job.[6]

Cubans had good reason to be wary. The U.S. Army arriving in Cuba in 1898, for example, was disgusted by the hit-and-run tactics of the Cuban Liberation Army—tactics that had allowed the outgunned, outprovisioned, and outnumbered insurgents to bring the colonial power of Spain to the very brink of collapse—and relegated the Cuban soldiers to the tasks of porters and guides. After presiding over the surrender of the Spanish forces at Santiago de Cuba, a victory due in no small part to yellow fever among the Spanish troops brought by Máximo Gómez's invincible General July, the United States claimed full credit for the liberation of Cuba and demanded Cubans' unconditional gratitude.[7]

With respect to public health, however, Delfín's concern appears misplaced. Cubans made up not only the rank-and-file of the army of street sweepers, garbage collectors, and Special Sanitation Brigade members employed by the Department of Sanitation in Havana but also their foremen and supervisors. Cubans similarly conducted the critical work of house inspections, and the commission of physicians tasked with identifying cases of yellow fever consisted of Major William C. Gorgas and three Cuban doctors: Carlos J. Finlay, Antonio Díaz Albertini, and Juan Guiteras. Finlay, in fact, was the president of the commission and was also the originator of the mosquito theory of yellow fever transmission that, when elaborated to include Henry Carter's period of extrinsic incubation and proven by the experiments of Jesse Lazear and Walter Reed, provided the basis for ridding the island of yellow fever. The many Cubans who had played such important parts in the initial public health successes of their new country knew themselves capable of continuing the work unaided. How they resisted the continuing U.S. discourse to the contrary is the subject of this chapter.

Fighting Mosquitoes, Fighting Hegemony

After the end of the second U.S. occupation in January 1909, Cuban officials knew well that maintaining a level of sanitation acceptable to the United States was critical to the independence of their young nation. "It may seem like a joke but it is nevertheless true that, if our Government neglects the persecution of the stegomyia mosquito and an epidemic of yellow fever results, our independence will be seriously compromised," one public health official observed.[8] The matter was not considered a joke at all. When Havana's garbage collectors and street sweepers went on strike in October 1909, Cuba's new secretary of state, Justo García Vélez, charged that Dr. Matías Duque, the secretary of health and charities, was not doing enough to bring the strike, the consequent risk of an outbreak of disease, and so the threat of another U.S. intervention to a quick end. The accusation led to "a serious altercation between the men," and Duque challenged García Vélez to a duel. Seconds were named, but at that point President José Miguel Gómez stepped in to resolve the dispute between the two members of his cabinet. García Vélez was ultimately removed from office over the incident.[9]

Despite the manifest seriousness with which Cubans took issues of sanitation, U.S. newspapers and professional journals maintained an image of Cubans as unwilling or unable to fulfill the public health obligations imposed on them by the Platt Amendment to the Cuban constitution. One highly respected medical journal, the *Medical Record*, painted a picture of irresponsible politicians and declining sanitary conditions in Cuba. Cuban lawmakers, the journal's editor opined, are "so shortsighted as not to see that the prosperity of the island, and consequently a full treasury for personal needs, depends upon keeping their country in a sanitary condition and so attractive to tourists and settlers, in a matter that concerns themselves." Yellow fever lurked in hidden corners of the island, he claimed, and cases of the disease continued to be misdiagnosed by Cuban doctors. Only an unceasing fight against mosquitoes would prevent yellow fever from again becoming endemic in Havana, but there was "unfortunately little reason to hope" that the Cubans would continue this fight. The *Record,* like other U.S. observers, was concerned not primarily with the health of the island, but rather the threat that conditions in Cuba would pose to the United States. The Cubans, its editor argued, "may sink their island to the level of Haiti, if they please, but it is intolerable that they should suffer conditions to be renewed in Havana which endanger the health and prosperity of our entire Gulf Coast." There was only one logical conclusion to be drawn, according to the editorial:

> The United States government may let the Gomez administration run Cuba as it will, waste its resources, pile up an unpayable debt, and put an end to public improvements, but that Havana can be allowed to become again a pest hole and a menace to the lives and the property of our own citizens is unthinkable. . . . [O]ur government should take the matter in its own hands.[10]

This view was common. A writer to the *Boston Transcript* commented on the decline in sanitation he claimed he had witnessed in Havana:

> When the American soldiery was withdrawn from the island a year or more ago Cuba was as clean as a whistle. Yellow fever had been wiped out and cholera was a thing of the past. Two years ago one could sit out in the parks or loll in the chairs in front of the hotels in comfort. To-day the mosquitos [*sic*] would eat one up. When the United States was in control, Cuba could give lessons in cleanliness to most American cities. To-day, it is said, one needs to be guided only by the nostrils to find the great market in Havana.[11]

The *New York Times* argued that the Gómez administration, like that of Estrada Palma after the first intervention, was negligent in its public health efforts, "with the practical certainty that before long there will be a recurrence of yellow fever in Havana, with all its consequent danger to the neighboring cities in the United States." Officials in the U.S. State Department, the paper reported, considered the stalled progress of sanitary improvements to be proof that Cubans were "congenitally incapable of adapting themselves to the restraints of successful government." If the Cubans continued to behave so irresponsibly in matters of sanitation, another intervention would no doubt result:

> The authority of the United States to intervene in Cuba under the so-called "Platt Amendment" to the Constitution is unquestioned. . . . The Taft Administration is keeping close watch on developments in the island and is hopeful of avoiding another smash. But it is admitted that there are grounds for no little anxiety in the way Gomez is conducting affairs.[12]

Similar charges appeared in a 1910 editorial of the *Army and Navy Journal,* the "Gazette of the Regular and Volunteer Forces" since the U.S. Civil War. Tropical people were as a rule unconcerned with cleanliness, the editors wrote, and, but for the U.S. military, the Cubans never would have eradicated yellow fever:

> How quickly the people of the tropics drop back into conditions of apathy in matters of sanitation is shown in the case of Cuba, which supplies a striking illustration of the fact that the military system of sanitation employed by the American Army in the first and second occupations of the island was the only thing that would have rid Cuba of the yellow fever and other diseases. . . . It was the bayonet behind the sanitary regulations of the military governors that alone did that.[13]

With the withdrawal of U.S. troops, sanitation efforts in Cuba came to an end, the *Journal* asserted: Neither the efforts of U.S. advisor to the Sanitary Department, Jefferson R. Kean, to provide Cuba with sanitary laws that were a model for the world nor the success of the provisional government's fight against yellow fever "could give the Cubans the will or the ability to live up to those high standards of sanitation and cleanliness."[14] Produced and reproduced by articles such as these, the prevalent view in the United States was that Cubans were a dirty people and only close U.S. supervision would prevent Cuba from again becoming a haven for disease.

This discourse did not go unchallenged, however. Cubans— particularly public health officials—refused to be characterized as irresponsible, dirty, and dependent on the United States in sanitary matters. Rather than accept claims that could serve as grounds for another U.S. invasion of Cuba, they insisted that the island was then and would always remain free of yellow fever through Cubans' own efforts. Duque, the duel-fighting secretary of health and charities, blasted the *Medical Record* for its claims that public health was being mismanaged and neglected on the island. "The administration of President Gómez will be as just, as equitable, as wise, as orderly and as methodic, as that of General Wood, whom we never forget, and as that of the Hon. Mr. Magoon," he wrote. "We may firmly assure that . . . the persecution of the mosquito is carried on at present just as it was by Colonel Kean" during the second intervention.[15] There was no possibility that yellow fever could be misdiagnosed in Cuba, he argued, since those in charge of yellow fever investigations were internationally recognized as the world's foremost experts on the disease: Juan Guiteras, Carlos Finlay, and Arístides Agramonte. Their many years of experience with yellow fever and the diseases with which it was often confused ensured that there would be no mistakes in diagnosis.[16] Moreover, the proper procedure for discerning the symptoms of yellow fever was widely disseminated to the doctors on the island. Yellow fever could not exist in Cuba, Duque insisted:

> Our means of defense, our system of house inspection, not only in the urban districts but in the rural as well, give us sufficient security to permit us to state, even in an emphatic manner, the absolute impossibility that yellow fever should exist, and much less that it should take hold of us to the extent of making Cuba a dangerous territory to the United States, our great and good friend. We seek to maintain healthy conditions, not merely for the benefit of the United States, but for the welfare of our own country.[17]

U.S. sanitarians who had seen the Cuban arrangements firsthand agreed that they were exemplary, Duque noted. He quoted the president of the Louisiana State Board of Health, who said of the Cuban board of yellow fever experts: "This Commission seems to be a splendid institution, and it would be an admirable thing, could it be possible, for every Southern State to supervise its contagious diseases as closely and thoroughly as does Cuba."[18] Contrary to the story of Cuban indifference repeatedly told in the United States, Duque maintained that "with respect to Sanitation we have the greatest desire to maintain such excellent conditions that all the nations of the world will envy us."[19]

Juan Guiteras, who held the post of chief sanitary officer of Havana during the Gómez administration, also refuted the assertions of Cuban sanitary neglect that pervaded discussions of the island in the United States. He railed against the fact that "every recurring year, at the beginning of the tourist season, some paper or papers in the United States start this same ball rolling. It grows through repetition of the statement, and is taken up at last by important publications." In response to the *Army and Navy Journal,* Guiteras recounted Cuba's sanitary accomplishments and demanded some answers:

> What facts have you . . . upon which to base your statements? Is it that we have less typhoid fever than most of your cities? . . . Is it that we have managed to keep smallpox out of our territory, though we are in communication with your States, where the disease prevails? . . . Is it that we are maintaining at great expense a system of inspections all over the island for the destruction of larvae?

"As for the people sitting out in the parks and lolling in chairs in front of the hotels, free from the annoyance of mosquitoes, in the days of the intervention," he continued, "I may assure the tourists who will come to Cuba that the conditions are now the same, or perhaps better, than they were during the intervention." Cubans would not sit idly by while U.S. observers defamed their hard-earned achievements in public health, Guiteras wrote: "We must give the facts as they are when we find that they are constantly being disfigured and misinterpreted. As to the debt we owe the United States for enabling us to bring about these results, we can only repay it by doing precisely what you are not willing to concede that we are doing—maintaining the standard."[20]

The Cuban doctors struggled to counter the barrage of U.S. claims that only the United States could prevent Cuba from again becoming a source of contagious disease. Guiteras informed the readers of the *Medical Record* that, far from neglecting public health, the Cuban government had allocated four million dollars for its protection. Cubans, he wrote, were "consolidating and broadening at the same time the operations in Preventive Medicine that were started during the American intervention."[21] The United States, during its two occupations of the island, had greatly advanced sanitation in Cuba, Guiteras conceded, but the Cubans were fully capable of handling the issue on their own.

Matías Duque, Guiteras's colleague, agreed. The Cuban government, he repeatedly declared, made sanitation a priority of the highest importance:

> Our current sanitary state is one of the best in the world. The sanitary laws created by Colonel Kean and established by the

Honorable Governor Magoon, are reaching every day new tri-
umphs, as can be observed by looking at the monthly statistics, where one can see the diminishment of deaths by trans-
missible diseases. Those practices are continued with exquisite
vigilance, as President Gómez's government gives preference to
conserving and ameliorating everyday more the sanitation of
the Republic.[22]

In addition to keeping the island free of yellow fever, Duque pointed out,
the Gómez government had also made important advances in tuberculosis, leprosy, waterworks in the cities, and tropical medicine in general, benefiting not only the Cubans, but also the people of the United
States.[23] The current Cuban administration was doing its job well, "not
to say that this has been better than the American administration, but to
affirm that if the Intervention left the administration in good condition,
the Cuban Government has made them better every day, basing it on the
law of perfection and not as the defamatory lie has wanted to portray us
before the civilized world."[24]

In its own publication, the Cuban National Board of Health and
Charities sought to demonstrate that Duque's claim of continual improvements was not empty rhetoric: nearly every volume contained de-
scriptions of the new and innovative techniques that were employed in
eradicating mosquitoes—and so the threat of yellow fever—from the
cities and towns of the island. One such innovation consisted of placing
small fish in water containers. In towns without waterworks, many residents continued to keep potable water in large barrels or clay vessels.
Although wooden barrels were easily covered or oiled and then fitted
with a spout for drawing water, the clay pots commonly used in many
areas could not be easily modified: sanitary crews attempting to place
a spigot on the clay reservoirs found that the containers would crack
easily, and the shape of the containers also prevented the installation of
removable lids. For these reasons, the Sanitary Department gave away
biajacas, a type of small fish that fed on mosquito larvae, to be kept in
the containers. In the constant attempt to find the most efficient variety
of fish for the purpose, the chief of sanitation of Camagüey exchanged
these fish for another type, *guajacones,* which were deemed both better
at eating the larvae and easier to keep.[25]

The sanitary authorities in Cuba also worked to show that they were
quickly adopting the latest advances in fumigation techniques. The covering of entire buildings with canvas rather than attempting to stop up
each crack and crevice with wadded paper, a new technique described

at the 1905 American Public Health Association meeting by the Mexican delegate, Eduardo Licéaga, was, the Cubans declared, employed to great effect in the Cuban campaign to destroy the mosquito. Cuban sanitarians described in detail how they had, in the course of applying this new method, experimented with different types and sizes of canvas to determine, given the type of building that needed fumigation, the best arrangement for each particular case.[26]

Cuban sanitation officials also sought to demonstrate that they dealt with any suspected cases of yellow fever quickly and appropriately. Guiteras documented the Cuban response when three workers were admitted with a fever to the United Fruit Company Hospital. First, the Cuban doctors informed sanitary authorities in the United States. "I claim that you can not properly meet such an emergency if you pretend to hide things. As soon as we had, therefore, confirmation from competent authority to the effect that one of the cases might be accepted as yellow fever, at least for the purpose of sanitary measures, we made it known to our neighbors that we were busy with this trouble," Guiteras explained.[27] The same day that the cases were reported, the Health Department sent two doctors with yellow fever expertise along with ten experienced men of the disinfection brigade and all the equipment necessary to treat the premises. They arrived in Banes the following evening, and by the next morning they fumigated the workers' barracks with the assistance of the local health officer and his five employees. Three days later, following extensive observation and examination, the suspected cases were determined not to be yellow fever at all but rather malaria.[28] There could be no doubt that Cuban sanitarians were perfectly capable of handling a suspected outbreak of yellow fever without U.S. assistance.

Cuban officials and health authorities knew well the importance of sanitation to both the health *and* the independence of their country and worked diligently to maintain the highest possible standards. Observers in the United States nevertheless justified the continuing domination of Cuba by depicting Cubans as dirty, irresponsible, and incapable of managing their own public health. Cuban sanitarians refused to accept this account, struggled to refute it, and so denied U.S. domination the legitimacy that Cuban dependence would provide.

Dependence Exposed

Cuban public health officials knew that rather than Cuba being dependent on the United States, the relationship was actually the reverse. They knew—and declared to the world—that while Cuba pursued the politically difficult and costly measures of mosquito eradication, the United States neglected these same measures in its southern cities. Far from perceiving the sanitation of the island as the benefit of U.S. domination that legitimated the unequal relationship between the two countries, Cubans recognized that the United States had dominated Cuban public health policy to provide benefits to its own economy and citizens.

Juan Guiteras repeatedly decried the fact that the citizens of the United States took their country's occupation and reoccupation of Cuba as proof that Cubans could teach them nothing about maintaining public health and preventing yellow fever. "It is very regrettable that the special circumstances that affect our country," he wrote, "prevent the full appreciation of the lessons taught by the three years (1905–1908) of the recent visit of our ancient enemy, the so-called Antillean disease. In fact, everything that happens in Cuba is seen, from abroad, through the prism of suspicions awakened by conflicting interests that are not always of the best character."[29]

The continuing, but misplaced, concern expressed in both the popular press and professional publications of the United States that Cuba was dirty and that Cubans needed to work harder to clean up the island to avoid threatening the U.S. South with yellow fever, Guiteras observed, only underscored the reality that U.S. sanitarians had failed to learn and adopt the measures that were the foundation of Cuban success in controlling yellow fever: the immediate reporting of all suspected yellow fever cases and the unrelenting campaign against mosquitoes.[30] Sanitary authorities in the U.S. South, he pointed out, continued to rely solely on the use of quarantines against infected ports to avoid the spread of yellow fever and only activated antimosquito work in the course of an outbreak. Cubans knew that only constant attention to the eradication of mosquitoes was truly effective: "I hope," Guiteras wrote, "that the names and works of Gorgas, Kean and other medical officers of your Army will be appreciated as they are here."[31]

Arístides Agramonte, who had worked closely with Finlay, Reed, Gorgas, and Kean and then became a professor of bacteriology at the University of Havana, drew similar conclusions. At medical conferences and in the pages of medical journals, he recounted not only how much the constant threat of Cuba's powerful neighbor to the north had contributed to the excellent sanitary knowledge and condition of the island but also how sharply the Cuban public health situation contrasted with that of the United States. Before the assembled experts at the Sixteenth International Medical Congress in Budapest in 1909, he declared that his purpose was "to bring out before this Congress in an unmistakable manner, how much better we are prepared than any of the other nations of the American continents to encounter and defeat yellow fever, since from a sanitary point of view we have been the cynosure of all eyes and our reputation in this respect has been maligned upon more than one occasion."[32]

After a careful consideration of the different measures the Cuban sanitary authorities had enacted on the island, Agramonte denounced the United States for its lack of efforts against yellow fever, "since, as I have said, from a sanitary standpoint we have been in the public eye for several years, I cannot refrain from calling the attention of my hearers to the superiority of our organization when compared with that of our neighboring countries." The United States, he declared,

> and more especially the States bordering on the Gulf of Mexico, depend almost exclusively upon quarantine measures to prevent the introduction of yellow fever; their towns are overrun by stegomyia mosquitos [sic]; the city of New Orleans, in Louisiana, which depends for its water supply upon the use of cisterns in every house, has failed to keep them all properly covered, and mosquitos [sic] are to-day nearly as plentiful as before the dreadful epidemic of 1905. The nonimmune population is widely disseminated and in the hand of private practitioners, who will fail to recognize the first cases, or will hide them, as they did in the memorable summer of 1905. The same may be said of the other Southern States whose bugbear is yellow fever and whose protective mainstay is quarantine, the least useful measure which may be implanted in any country for its defense against said infection.[33]

Even Mexico was doing more to fight yellow fever than the United States, Agramonte noted. In Veracruz, the Mexican sanitary authorities routinely conducted house-to-house inspections, dispatched oiling brigades, and employed the other techniques perfected in Havana.[34] The United States was not spending the money or political capital necessary to prevent yellow fever from gaining a foothold in its cities, Agramonte told his audience; rather, the United States relied solely on the efforts of the Cubans to keep the region free of the disease.

Cuban public health officials were not the only ones to recognize that keeping the island free of yellow fever was primarily a benefit to the United States. Ordinary Cubans were well aware that they rarely fell

victim to the disease and therefore that the heroic efforts of Cuba's Department of Public Health were expended, in the words of one Cuban
newspaper editor, to "prevent the disease that may affect the foreigner
and more specifically the one of American nationality," while there had
been little or no progress against tuberculosis, the disease that continued to kill more Cubans than any other.[35] Indeed, many Cubans felt that
the current work of the department was a complete waste of money and
so engaged in "passive resistance and ironic indifference towards all
sanitary measures, causing in that way even greater difficulties" for the
island's doctors and sanitarians.[36]

The public health situation in Cuba was incontrovertibly better after
a decade of U.S. domination of the island's sanitation policies than it
had been under Spanish rule. The doctors, public health officials, and
citizens of Cuba knew, however, that the great expense and personal
impositions they endured to maintain the sanitary conditions insisted
upon by the United States served principally to protect southern U.S.
port cities from yellow fever—cities that undertook little or no efforts
to improve their own sanitation in order to protect themselves. Under
these circumstances, public health could not provide legitimacy to the
U.S. domination of the island.

Recovering Finlay's Glory

Public health officials, doctors, and other observers in the United States
placed all of the blame for yellow fever on Cubans and insisted that
Cuba alone bear the burdens of fighting it, yet they were quick to claim
for the United States the full credit for the scientific understanding of
how the disease was spread. Just as Cubans struggled against the U.S.
characterization of Cuba as inherently dirty and disease-ridden and
fought to make known that the United States was dependent on Cuba
for public health rather than the reverse, they refused to accept U.S.
mythmaking regarding the scientific victory over yellow fever and insisted on acknowledging and celebrating the important role of their
compatriot, Dr. Carlos J. Finlay, in the story.

By early 1902, yellow fever had been eliminated in Cuba. This triumph of public health was made possible by scientific advancements
in knowledge of the disease. Carlos Finlay's theory that yellow fever
was transmitted not by general filth or infected objects but only by
the bite of an infected mosquito had been conclusively proven by experiments conducted by the U.S. Yellow Fever Commission headed by
Walter Reed. Despite Finlay's central role, the prevalent account of the

conquest of yellow fever in the United States ignored or belittled the fundamental contribution made by the Cuban doctor in deducing the relationship between mosquitoes and the disease. This tendency began with Reed himself.

Although Jesse Lazear had pursued Finlay's mosquito theory at the suggestion of Henry Rose Carter, and with no involvement on Reed's part, Reed was quick to claim credit for Lazear's discoveries when Lazear died in the course of his work. On the very day that Lazear succumbed to yellow fever, Reed claimed for the first time that, "from the beginning of our work, I have insisted on the common sense theory of an intermediate host, such as the mosquito, being the carrier of the parasite of y[ellow] fever."[37] Despite his absence from Cuba during Lazear's experiments, Reed quickly became known as the great organizing mind of all of the work done by the members of the Yellow Fever Commission; Lazear, according to this account, had merely been an assistant following Reed's instructions. Given his unwillingness to give due credit to his own fallen colleague, it is no surprise that Reed refused to recognize the even more fundamental contributions of Carlos Finlay. He chastised William C. Gorgas, chief sanitary officer of Havana during the first occupation, for crediting Finlay with originating the mosquito theory, bemoaning the attribution as an attempt to "honey buggle the simpering old idiot." Gorgas denied the charge: "I think [Finlay] is an old trump as modest as he is kindly & true. His reasoning for selecting the Stegomyia as the bearer of yellow fever is the best piece of logical reasoning that can be found in medicine anywhere."[38] Despite Gorgas's arguments, most U.S. observers followed Reed and gave Finlay little or no credit for inferring the mosquito theory of yellow fever transmission.

Cubans, however, rejected U.S. accounts that removed their compatriot Finlay from the story of the triumph over yellow fever. "There exists undoubtedly some tendency in the United States to diminish the importance of the work of Dr. Finlay in the foundation of these new doctrines," Guiteras wrote in 1910, but Finlay "participates in equal terms, as I see it, in the great glory of the discovery, taking away, naturally, the character of a solely American triumph." Finlay alone maintained that mosquitoes carried yellow fever, Guiteras pointed out; he was "the only man who, between 1898 and 1900 could say and do these things. The only man in that moment, as in all the previous history of this issue, was this great Antillean . . . he combined in his fertile brain the faculties of his ancestors; the persistent and logical reasoning of the Scottish, with the lively imagination of the French."[39]

Finlay, according to Cuban observers, could not be allowed to suffer the fate that befell many great innovators. At first, the Cuban sanitarian José Manuel Espin noted, the prevailing opinion often criticizes new discoveries, and their originators are considered eccentric. Then, as knowledge of the finding diffuses, the discoverer is ridiculed and "made the object of rude remarks." Finally, when the merit of the discovery at last becomes apparent, it is attributed to someone else. "This is what has happened with the modern doctrine about the transmission of certain diseases by the mosquito, particularly that which refers to yellow fever," Espin wrote. "The tendency is to take away all the glory of our Finlay."[40] Cubans, however, would continue to hold up his accomplishments, "and so, as much as it is attempted to take away the glory of the founder of the modern doctrine, grateful posterity, making justice, will dedicate preferential place in the pages of the History of Medicine" to Finlay.[41]

Cuban public health officials refused to acquiesce to the distortion of the historical record. When one U.S. doctor published an article recounting the "scientific conquest of yellow fever" that introduced the work of Reed's commission in Havana with the observation that "some had already suspected that the mosquito had something to do with yellow fever," the officials of the Cuban National Board of Health and Charities reprinted the item in full in their journal.[42] They explained:

> Leaving aside the many historical inexactitudes, scientific errors, and false statements that abound in that work, we wanted to take advantage of the opportunity to give it space in our columns to demonstrate one more time the irrationality and ingratitude with which foreigners, save a few exceptions, leave completely forgotten our compatriots to whom the discovery and confirmation of the transmission of yellow fever by the stegomyia mosquito is principally owed. In Dr. Paulsor's unfortunate article he does not even mention the names of Finlay, Agramonte, and Guiteras.[43]

As observers in the United States and beyond again and again neglected to acknowledge the important roles played by Cubans in the defeat of yellow fever, again and again Cubans would have to correct them. "Fortunately," the Cuban sanitarians argued, "the light of truth always clears out the underbrush, and the glory that properly pertains to our countrymen is founded in support as firm as the extinction of yellow fever in Cuba and a great part of the Americas."[44]

Persistent claims to the contrary, however, continued to obscure what Cubans viewed as the obvious importance of Finlay's work to the triumph over yellow fever. At the Congreso de la Prensa Médica Latina in 1927, José A. López del Valle, secretary of the Cuban National Board of Health and Charities and a professor of sanitation and hygiene at the School of Medicine of the University of Havana, addressed the assembled delegates on the injustice of the situation and the Cuban resolve to correct it:

> Ignored by some, attempted to be denied by others, pretended to be obscured by many, the glory belongs to Dr. Carlos J. Finlay, of Cuba, for discovering the means of transmission of Yellow Fever, fixing the basis for its prophylaxis, and being the first in enunciating a scientific doctrine about the transmission of illnesses from "man to man" through an intermediary agent; we consider it proper to take advantage of the celebration of this congress as well as all the meetings of scientific character celebrated throughout the world, until [these] scientific truths . . . are recognized in a clear and definite manner by all.[45]

Jorge Le-Roy, secretary of the Academy of Medical, Physical, and Natural Sciences of Havana, was determined to expose those most responsible for deprecating Finlay's legacy. He condemned "the obstinate persistence with which the Rockefeller Foundation over many years has attributed to Reed and the Commission named by the American Government that he headed (1900–1901) the *discovery of the method of transmission of yellow fever*" and he blasted the editors of the *Journal of the American Medical Association* for repeatedly making "statements as categorical as they are unjustified, which it is not possible to pass by without correcting, such as, 'Twenty-one years ago, the United States commission headed by Walter Reed discovered in Havana the method of transmission (of yellow fever).'"[46] After reviewing that it was Finlay who had elaborated the mosquito theory of yellow fever transmission in 1881, two decades before the work of the U.S. Yellow Fever Commission of Walter Reed, Le-Roy leveled his judgment:

> There has been sin either by crass ignorance or by a manifest determination to usurp the glory of the biggest man that America has produced on the field of medicine in the past half century. If it is because of the first, we must advise that this ignorance is unacceptable in those who occupy elevated positions in the

scientific world. If it is the second, the full weight of the condemning censure of those who love the truth and justice should fall upon them.[47]

Cuban observers worked tenaciously to discredit the narrative of the scientific triumph over yellow fever prevalent in the United States and elsewhere that excluded Finlay and accorded all credit to U.S. scientists. The eradication of yellow fever from Cuba was not a gift bestowed by a benevolent United States for which Cubans should be grateful, they maintained, but rather a shared enterprise in which Cubans, most notably Finlay, had made contributions at least equal to those of the U.S. Yellow Fever Commission. The success of the fight against yellow fever in Cuba could not be attributed to the United States alone, and therefore this success could not serve to justify the U.S. domination of the island.

To many Cubans, the link between insisting that Finlay receive credit for his role in the fight against yellow fever and maintaining an independent Cuba unbowed by U.S. domination was not merely implicit. At the 1911 meeting of the Academy of Medical, Physical, and Natural Sciences of Havana, the assembled scientists celebrated Finlay as a Cuban national champion equal to the heroes of the struggle for independence. Guiteras argued that Finlay, by discovering that yellow fever was transmitted by the stegomyia mosquito, was the Cuban who had, "by universal judgment, raised highest the name of Cuba."[48]

"The independence of nations, it has been said, lies not in the rifles of their soldiers, but in the spirit of their citizens," observed Juan Santos Fernández. "The sons of Cuba who first fought to obtain a nation . . . stayed true to that singular flag, but there were many who saw in the foreign domination that would one day supplant Spain an easier way to profit from their own soil." Finlay, despite his years of education in France and the United States, had always remained steadfastly Cuban. According to Santos Fernández, Finlay always "felt with fervent emotion for his free and independent homeland and gave himself completely to it with his glory and exceptional greatness."[49] His accomplishments on behalf of Cuba must not be forgotten, Santos Fernández exhorted his audience: "we must work ceaselessly to not allow the fire of recognition in our hearts to extinguish and to maintain it always alive."[50] Recalling Finlay's achievements was more than appropriate. For them, as Cubans, it was a patriotic duty.[51]

The association between Finlay and the new Cuban nation only grew stronger in the years after his death in 1915. At the dedication of a bronze plaque in the great lecture hall of the University of Havana in 1927, López del Valle claimed that it would be an insult to his audience to narrate the Cuban doctor's accomplishments; all of those present were entirely familiar with them. The same was not true, however, in other countries, especially the United States, López del Valle lamented: "In text books, official reports of scientific institutions, in professional and political newspapers, when dealing with yellow fever prophylaxis, of its propagation, of the successes obtained in its control, either the name of the brilliant Cuban is silenced, or the discovery is attributed to other entities."[52] Any mention of Finlay, he complained, was made only in passing; in foreign scientific centers and academies "it has been necessary that the Cuban Delegates reclaim for Finlay all the glory that is properly his for his brilliant accomplishments."[53]

"For Cubans," López del Valle argued, "it is a duty and a debt of honor to give recognition to all that is owed to Finlay, his wonderful discovery, his immortal experiences, and his persevering and original works."[54] He called for more projects like the foundation, by the secretary of sanitation, of the new Finlay Institute, "a 'living document,' an 'animated monument' to his memory that, with the works, investigations, and teachings that will be realized in it and their benefits to humanity and Science, progress and national culture, will be like an eternal hymn sung throughout the ages to the glory of Finlay."[55] Similar efforts to memorialize Finlay must be carried out abroad, López del Valle urged. Cuban legations and consulates had already begun distributing copies of Finlay's works to the various academies of science, libraries, newspapers, publishers, and scientific centers across Europe so that all could become familiar with the importance of his scientific achievements. To champion Finlay against those who would forget him was a duty for all Cubans, López del Valle stressed: "Let us be clear that we must faithfully undertake these steps, not only to establish a true principal for the name of Finlay, but also for our Cuba, from which no one can strip its proper glories!"[56]

In the eyes of many Cubans, Finlay's scientific contributions to the eradication of yellow fever symbolized all of the contributions of Cubans to the creation of their new independent nation. If the United States obliterated Finlay's identification of the mosquito as the transmitter of yellow fever and claimed for its own scientists the accomplishment, then all Cubans' efforts on behalf of their country would certainly be forgotten as well. To vindicate the glory of Finlay was to vindicate an independent Cuba; just as U.S. attempts to monopolize credit for the defeat of yellow fever were unfounded, the continuing U.S. domination of the island was unjust and illegitimate. Cubans would accept neither.

: : :

The second occupation of Cuba by U.S. troops had made clear to Cuban officials that sanitation to prevent yellow fever was a national priority critical to the sovereignty of their young republic, and their efforts successfully ensured that the disease never again appeared on the island. The discourse surrounding the triumph over yellow fever, however, was sharply contested for decades afterward. Observers in the United States sought to justify U.S. domination of Cuba by depicting Cubans as a dirty, irresponsible people who cared little if their island became a haven for infectious disease. Advancements of U.S. scientists alone had made the elimination of yellow fever in Cuba possible, these observers insisted, and close U.S. supervision alone would ensure that the dreaded disease did not return to the island from which it had so long threatened the ports of the U.S. South.

Cubans refused to accept this account. Determined to avoid any grounds for U.S. intervention, Cuban public health officials repeatedly refuted U.S. claims of declining conditions in Cuba and demonstrated that their sanitation efforts in the years after 1909 employed the very latest techniques and maintained the very highest standards. They denied attempts to legitimate U.S. domination on the grounds that Cuba was dependent on the United States in matters of sanitation. The truth, they argued with considerable justification, was that the United States was dependent on Cuba to keep yellow fever from infecting the filthy cities of the U.S. South, where even rudimentary sanitary measures were neglected. Moreover, Cubans rejected the view that the knowledge of how to defeat yellow fever was a gift to Cuba from the United States; they demanded that the United States and the world acknowledge the contributions of their countrymen, especially Carlos J. Finlay, to the scientific conquest of yellow fever. Just as the quick victory of the U.S. Army over Spanish forces in Cuba was made possible by decades of struggle by Cuban independence fighters, the final confirmation by the U.S. Yellow Fever Commission that mosquitoes transmitted the disease was based on decades of persistent work by the Cuban doctor. In upholding Finlay, Cubans upheld their own independence from U.S. domination; in rejecting Reed as a lone scientific hero who had given the Cubans the secret to yellow fever, they rejected the United States as a protector they required to give them sustained sanitation and security from disease.

7 Conclusions

Diseases and the public health efforts to control them reveal relations of power. When some sicken and others remain healthy, the response demonstrates whose interests are considered and whose are ignored. Yellow fever in Havana had a decidedly different impact on Cubans than it did on the United States. Cubans suffered little from the disease itself; mild childhood infections provided most of them with lifetime immunity. In the southern United States, however, yellow fever epidemics that started in Havana wreaked havoc, killing by the thousands and snarling commerce for months on end. For U.S. influence to expand into the Caribbean and beyond, the disease had to be controlled at its source. That public health in Cuba focused on yellow fever and not the diseases that most afflicted Cubans illuminates U.S. domination over the island.

Yellow fever repeatedly spread from Havana to the U.S. South in the late nineteenth century, paralyzing the southern economy and in turn affecting the entire country. Even in the absence of an epidemic, the threat of yellow fever was a constant encumbrance to the U.S. economy. To protect against the introduction of the disease, state and federal government agencies had to enact quarantines that were not only expensive to enforce but also a disruption to the growing trade between the United

States and Cuba, as well as between different locales within the United States. This book has argued that a principal reason for the 1898 U.S. intervention in the war between Cuba and Spain was to alleviate conditions that threatened the U.S. South: the increase of yellow fever and the neglect of sanitary measures in Havana brought about by the war were intolerable.

Once the Spanish forces in Cuba were defeated and the U.S. military government of Cuba was established, controlling Havana's endemic yellow fever surfaced as a chief concern in governmental policies. U.S. officials and medical authorities expended great efforts in cleaning the city, focusing on eliminating filth, which they then believed to be the cause of the disease. When these efforts failed to check yellow fever, the government undertook increasingly frantic efforts.

The failure of the initial sanitary campaign heightened the need for a better understanding of the source of yellow fever. It was these circumstances that motivated the U.S. authorities to fund further research on the disease with the Yellow Fever Commission headed by Walter Reed. I have argued that, contrary to popular understandings today, the "discovery" of the mosquito vector for yellow fever initially happened without the knowledge of Walter Reed himself. It was the finding of Henry Rose Carter that yellow fever required nearly two weeks before spreading from initial infection to secondary cases that eventually drew the attention of Jesse Lazear of the U.S. Yellow Fever Commission to Carlos J. Finlay's theory that a mosquito was responsible for propagating yellow fever. Lazear kept his work secret from Reed until after he had become the first to succeed in experimentally transmitting the disease. When, after Lazear's death, Reed's experiments convincingly proved that mosquitoes alone transmitted the disease, U.S. sanitation authorities adopted new measures that focused on the elimination of the mosquito and successfully rid Cuba of yellow fever.

But the U.S. government knew that the country's southern ports would not remain safe if yellow fever returned to Cuba after U.S. forces left the island. As argued here, maintaining the island free of yellow fever became an essential condition for the realization of Cuban independence. The United States, therefore, exacted the promise that Cubans would keep the island free of yellow fever as one of the prerequisites for the U.S. withdrawal from the island in 1902. The fifth clause of the Platt Amendment to the Cuban constitution assured that Cubans would maintain the sanitary standards established during the occupation in order to prevent the spread of epidemic disease.

In the early years of their republic Cubans denied that yellow fever was becoming a problem on the island, a fact that heightened tensions with the United States. The importance of Cuban sanitation to the United States was again underscored when the U.S. Army occupied Cuba for a second time and the total elimination of yellow fever became a central pursuit of U.S. officials.

Although the United States maintained close supervision of the island to ensure that its interests in sanitation were respected, I have shown that Cubans did not accept the implication that they were incapable of managing their own public health affairs. Cuban doctors and sanitarians rejected the accusations from U.S. sources that their country was falling into disrepair and that sanitary standards were not being kept up. On the contrary, they pointed out to the world that the United States did not employ mosquito control efforts known to prevent yellow fever and instead relied on Cuban sanitary efforts to keep its own southern states free of the disease. Observers in the United States attempted to use the issue of public health to establish Cuban inferiority and legitimate U.S. domination, but Cubans could and did argue that their efforts were far superior to those undertaken by their neighbors to the north.

In this light, for Cubans the figures of Carlos Finlay and Walter Reed became, I have argued, embodiments of independence and domination, respectively. While Cubans recognized that the United States imposed conditions of domination in the arena of disease prevention, they fought for the recognition of their own achievements in that arena. Proclaiming the glory of Finlay for Cuba could be understood as the assertion of a position of prominence in the global competition for medical and biological knowledge at a time when Europeans dominated the growing field of tropical medicine. In this case, however, insisting on and pressing for the recognition of Carlos Finlay as the central figure who indentified the mosquito vector of yellow fever was a way for Cubans to declare their triumph and their independence from the United States despite being bound by the terms of the Platt Amendment.

In the early decades of the twentieth century, U.S. concerns for public health came to extend far beyond Cuba, but these concerns were driven by the same factors that motivated the efforts to disinfect Havana. Even after yellow fever was eliminated from the island, the disease continued to threaten the economy of the U.S. South. As U.S. interests in Latin America expanded to other areas where yellow fever was prevalent, and as Latin American governments worked to attract U.S. investment to their countries, sanitation again surfaced as a field of power negotiation. The construction and opening of the Panama Canal in 1914 and the trade routes that it made accessible to both the United States and

Cuba created new dangers of yellow fever contagion, and U.S. efforts to prevent the spread of the disease grew.

After the successful elimination of the disease in Cuba, Panama became the next front in the U.S. war against yellow fever. Controlling yellow fever in Panama was an absolute necessity to the completion of the canal; the massive, eighteen-year effort of the French Compagnie Universelle du Canal Interocéanique to cross the isthmus failed, among other reasons, because of tens of thousands of deaths from yellow fever among the company's workers. Moreover, the canal zone would have to remain free of the disease or traffic through the canal would quickly infect U.S. ports. When the United States took over the canal building effort in 1904, William C. Gorgas, the U.S. Army doctor who had succeeded in eliminating yellow fever in Havana, was appointed to oversee the public health aspects of the operation, prevent a recurrence of the disastrous French experience, and ensure that the completed canal would be safe for transit.[1]

But the fight against yellow fever in Panama did not go as easily as it had in Havana. "The provision of water in Panama was obtained from wells, cisterns and barrels in every yard," Gorgas wrote.

> We found that it was not possible to enforce the covering or destruction of these breeding places, as we did in Havana; but we soon saw that if we introduced a supply of water it would be less difficult to induce the people to eliminate their wells. This was done and in six months after the introduction of the water supply and with the continued enforcement of sanitary measures yellow fever was eradicated.[2]

Gorgas and his team of sanitarians, veterans of the fight in Cuba, ensured that the construction and operation of the Panama Canal—and so further U.S. commercial expansion—were not endangered by yellow fever.[3]

The opening of the Panama Canal in 1914 brought with it not only new trade routes and markets for commerce but also new places for yellow fever to take hold. The large nonimmune populations of the mosquito-ridden and generally unsanitary Asian ports that were now more accessible to the Caribbean and eastern United States would, observers feared, rapidly develop into new foci of endemic yellow fever if the disease was ever introduced. As was the case in Cuba, the principal concern was not the health of the people of Asia, but the renewed threat of infection such conditions would present to the United States.

As Wycliff Rose, director of the International Health Commission of the Rockefeller Foundation, explained,

> the opening of the Panama Canal and the changing of trade relations resulting therefrom have given rise to widespread apprehension that yellow fever may be introduced into the Orient; and that once endemic in these densely populated regions it would become a permanent menace to the rest of the world.[4]

At the urging of Gorgas, then the surgeon general of the U.S. Army, in July 1914 the Rockefeller Foundation set out to eliminate yellow fever throughout the Americas.[5] The first target was to be Guayaquil, the principal port city of Ecuador. Guayaquil was the only site where yellow fever was endemic on the Pacific coast of South America; once the disease was defeated there, it would soon disappear from the other cities and towns of the coast.[6] Gorgas had visited the city in 1913 as the first part of a U.S. government effort to remove this new threat that the Panama Canal was about to link to the ports of the U.S. South. There would be no quick fix, he warned: although the circumstances in Guayaquil were much like those present in Havana in 1900, the success achieved in Cuba occurred under U.S. military rule and with the military governor's complete support. The sanitation efforts would be unlikely to receive such unconditional backing from the government in Ecuador, Gorgas noted, and it went without saying that U.S. troops would not be put at the disposal of the sanitation effort, a step that was not taken even in Panama. For these reasons, Gorgas concluded "that the situation in Guayaquil is more similar to that of Panama than to that of Havana, and that, as in the former place, it is not possible to give the sanitary officials sufficient authority to eradicate yellow fever without the aid of a water supply, paving, and sewerage."[7]

With the assistance of the Rockefeller Foundation and the support of the Ecuadorian government, however, this costly work was eventually completed. A new water supply and sewerage system were installed by 1916.[8] Although World War I delayed the full-scale antimosquito campaign until 1918, the regular house-to-house inspections would succeed in ending yellow fever in Guayaquil by the end of 1919.[9]

But the disease continued to persist in the region. In June 1918 there was a yellow fever epidemic in Guatemala. The next year outbreaks of the disease were reported in Peru, Brazil, Honduras, El Salvador, Nicaragua, and Mexico. Yellow fever was again epidemic in Peru in 1920. Cases were reported in Colombia in 1923. These outbreaks underscored that U.S. trade and investment in the region remained vulnerable to yellow fever, and the Rockefeller Foundation soon had programs in all of the countries vulnerable to the disease. Even the Brazilian government, which had succeeded in controlling yellow fever epidemics in Rio de Janeiro through the efforts of sanitarian Oswaldo Cruz, acquiesced to an expedition by the U.S. doctors of the Rockefeller Foundation to work in the Amazon areas afflicted by the disease. Although yellow fever was never eradicated from the Americas—the disease infected monkeys and could be conveyed by mosquitoes common in the Amazon, and so would remain dangerous in remote areas from eastern Panama to southern Brazil—it was at last brought well under control.[10]

The sanitary efforts undertaken in the Americas by the Rockefeller Foundation were only an extension of the self-interested public health endeavors carried out by the U.S. occupation government of Cuba. Eliminating endemic yellow fever in Guayaquil, for example, was no doubt beneficial to the Ecuadorian economy, but the principal goal of these efforts, like those in Havana, was to remove the threat to the continued economic expansion of the United States in the world.

: : :

The critical role of yellow fever in the formulation of the relationship between Cuba and the United States as described in this book raises some difficult questions. Why have historians so long neglected the public health component of U.S.-Cuban relations? How could generations of scholars have read the sanitation clause of the Platt Amendment without giving its implications a second thought?

The answers reside, I contend, in common conceptions of disease and health. Sanitation and the eradication of diseases are easily understood to be inherently desirable, to be unalloyed benefits to both individuals and a society. By targeting disease, government officials, doctors, and sanitary inspectors bring health. It is easy, upon finding that the U.S. occupation government of Cuba eliminated yellow fever on the island, to assume that this action was beneficial, first and foremost, to Cubans. After all, to be diseased is to suffer, and to end disease is to help.

The success of the U.S. occupation in eliminating yellow fever in Cuba and the conditions imposed in the Platt Amendment to ensure that Cuba remained sanitary are therefore quickly perceived as valuable actions that are intrinsically beneficial to Cubans, manifest evidence of U.S. benevolence toward the island's inhabitants. Characterizing the U.S. fight against yellow fever in this way, however, places it in the category of charitable work. As such, it may lead to an unpleasant perception of dependence but cannot be deemed a central aspect of the definition of U.S.-Cuban relations, certainly not as important as the overt political and economic restructuring of the island begun during the occupation and maintained under the Platt Amendment afterward.

Scholars, then, have looked at the Platt Amendment and, like the U.S. legislators who made the Cuban adoption of the measure mandatory for the U.S. withdrawal from the island, have not seen anything objectionable about a clause that requires that Cuba remain sanitary and healthy. The conditions imposed on the politics of the island, especially the provisions authorizing U.S. military intervention and a permanent U.S. naval presence, by contrast, are readily evident signs of the imposition of U.S. power over Cuba and, as such, have attracted a great deal of attention from historians in both Cuba and the United States. It is far less clear how ridding Cuba of disease and ostensibly securing a healthy future for its people could be an expression of U.S. interests and power, and therefore the subject has drawn little interest.

Nevertheless, the history of colonial public health demonstrates that government programs of sanitation and disease eradication in foreign countries are rarely simply charitable endeavors. The U.S. measures in Cuba were no exception. For decades, U.S. public health efforts revolved around first preventing the introduction of yellow fever to the southern United States from Havana and then putting an end to the threat to the South entirely by eliminating the disease in Cuba. The U.S. sanitation efforts in Cuba, in short, primarily served the interests of the United States, and Cubans resented this fact. Although public health has gone unnoticed and unrecognized by previous scholarship, any understanding of the U.S.-Cuban relationship during the late nineteenth and early twentieth centuries that neglects this dimension is incomplete. This book, then, opens an important avenue of understanding the events of that critical period in the history of the two countries.

                    : : :

Yellow fever had been a potent ally of the Cuban Liberation Army in its struggle to free the island from the Spanish empire; the disease, however, harmed not only the Spanish troops, but also the health and economy of the U.S. South. To protect the health of its citizens and its growing commercial interests, the United States responded by setting very definite limits to Cuban independence. With the loss of their one-time viral ally, Cubans struggled to overcome these limits alone.

Notes

CHAPTER I

1. This phrase is frequently attributed to Máximo Gómez, leader of the Cuban Liberation Army. See, for example, Manuel Moreno Fraginals, *Cuba/España, España/Cuba: Historia común* (Barcelona: Crítica, 1995), 250; Horatio Seymour Rubens, *Liberty: The Story of Cuba,* 2nd ed. (Salem: Ayer Publishing, 1970); John Lawrence Tone, *War and Genocide in Cuba, 1895–1898* (Chapel Hill: University of North Carolina Press, 2006), 75.

2. William C. Gorgas, *Report of Vital Statistics for the City of Havana for the Year 1901,* Miscellaneous Records of Various Agencies, 1899–1902, Records of the Military Government of Cuba, Record Group 140, National Archives, College Park, MD (hereafter MGC/ RG 140).

3. On prevalence of yellow fever in Havana before the British invasion, see Celia María Parcero Torre, *La pérdida de la Habana y las reformas borbónicas en Cuba, 1760–1773* (Valladolid: Junta de Castilla y León, Consejería de Educación y Cultura, 1998). As Parcero Torre revcals, the Spanish at that time counted on yellow fever to strike down the newly arrived British troops. On the African origins of the disease and its early history in the Caribbean, see Henry R. Carter, *Yellow Fever: An Epidemiological and Historical Study of Its Place of Origin* (Baltimore: Williams and Wilkins, 1931).

4. The U.S. experience with yellow fever has generated an extensive historiography. See, for example, John Duffy, *Sword of Pestilence: The New Orleans Yellow Fever Epidemic of 1853* (Baton Rouge: Louisiana State University Press, 1966);

Kahled J. Bloom, *The Mississippi Valley's Great Yellow Fever Epidemic of 1878* (Baton Rouge: Louisiana State University Press, 1993); Jo Ann Carrigan, *The Saffron Scourge: A History of Yellow Fever in Louisiana, 1796–1905* (Lafayette: Center for Louisiana Studies, University of Southwestern Louisiana, 1994); Margaret Humphreys, "Local Control Versus National Interest: The Debate over Southern Public Health, 1878–1884," *Journal of Southern History* 50, no. 3 (1984): 407–28; Humphreys, *Yellow Fever and the South* (Baltimore: Johns Hopkins University Press, 1992); John H. Ellis, *Yellow Fever and Public Health in the New South* (Lexington: University Press of Kentucky, 1992); James B. Speer, Jr., "Pestilence and Progress: Health Reform in Galveston and Houston during the Nineteenth Century," *Houston Review: History and Culture of the Gulf Coast* 2, no. 3 (1980): 120–32; Carrigan, "Privilege, Prejudice, and the Strangers' Disease in Nineteenth-Century New Orleans," *Journal of Southern History* 36, no. 4 (1970): 568–78; Edward Blum, "The Crucible of Disease: Trauma, Memory, and National Reconciliation during the Yellow Fever Epidemic of 1878," *Journal of Southern History* 69, no. 4 (2003): 791–820; William Coleman, *Yellow Fever in the North: The Methods of Early Epidemiology* (Madison: University of Wisconsin Press, 1987); John Harvey Powell, *Bring Out Your Dead: The Great Plague of Yellow Fever in Philadelphia in 1793* (New York: Arno Press, 1949; reprint, Philadelphia: University of Pennsylvania Press, 1993).

5. As Margaret Humphreys has observed, yellow fever was "above all a commercial problem, the control of which was essential to the development and prosperity of the South"; Humphreys, *Yellow Fever and the South,* 2.

6. Works focusing on these humanitarian impulses include Robert Endicott Osgood, *Ideals and Self-Interest in America's Foreign Relations: The Great Transformation of the Twentieth Century* (Chicago: University of Chicago Press, 1953); Frank Freidel, *The Splendid Little War* (Boston: Little Brown, 1958); Allan Keller, *The Spanish-American War: A Compact History* (New York: Hawthorn Books, 1969); David F. Trask, *The War with Spain in 1898* (New York: Macmillan, 1981). For the argument that such humanitarianism appealed to many men because chivalrously saving Cuba served to reinforce traditional gender roles in the face of growing challenges by women for political inclusion, see Kristin L. Hoganson, *Fighting for American Manhood: How Gender Politics Provoked the Spanish-American and Philippine-American Wars* (New Haven: Yale University Press, 1998).

7. See, for example, Jules R. Benjamin, *The United States and Cuba: Hegemony and Dependent Development, 1880–1934* (Pittsburgh: University of Pittsburgh Press, 1977); Benjamin, *The United States and the Origins of the Cuban Revolution: An Empire of Liberty in an Age of National Liberation* (Princeton: Princeton University Press, 1990); Philip S. Foner, *The Spanish-Cuban-American War and the Birth of American Imperialism, 1895–1902,* 2 vols. (New York: Monthly Review Press, 1972); Louis A. Pérez, Jr., *Cuba and the United States: Ties of Singular Intimacy* (Athens: University of Georgia Press, 1990); Pérez, *The War of 1898: The United States and Cuba in History and Historiography* (Chapel Hill: University of North Carolina Press, 1998). On the growing appreciation among U.S. officials of the military-strategic

importance of Cuba, see David F. Healy, *U.S. Expansionism: The Imperialist Urge in the 1890s* (Madison: University of Wisconsin Press, 1970), 22–28.

8. Diego Armus, ed., *Disease in the History of Latin America: From Malaria to AIDS* (Durham: Duke University Press, 2003); Marcos Cueto, *Salud, cultura y sociedad en América Latina* (Lima: Instituto de Estudios Peruanos, 1996); Cueto, *The Return of Epidemics: Health and Society in Peru during the Twentieth Century* (Aldershot, UK: Ashgate Publishing, 2001); César A. Mena and Fernando E. Cobelo, *Historia de la medicina en Cuba*, 2 vols. (Miami: Ediciones Universal, 1992); Consuelo Naranjo Orovio and Armando García González, *Medicina y racismo en Cuba: La ciencia ante la inmigración canaria en el siglo XX* (La Laguna, Tenerife: Centro de la Cultura Popular Canaria, 1996); Steven Palmer, *From Popular Medicine to Medical Populism: Doctors, Healers, and Public Power in Costa Rica, 1800–1940* (Durham: Duke University Press, 2003); Julyan G. Peard, *Race, Place, and Medicine* (Durham: Duke University Press, 1999); Pedro M. Pruna Goodgall, *Ciencia y científicos en Cuba colonial, La Real Academia de Ciencias de La Habana* (Havana: Editorial Academia, 2001); Benito Narey Ramos Domínguez and Jorge Adereguía Henríquez, *Medicina social y salud pública en Cuba* (Havana: Editorial Pueblo y Educación, 1990).

9. Marcos Cueto, "Sanitation from Above: Yellow Fever and Foreign Intervention in Peru, 1919–1922," *Hispanic American Historical Review* 72, no. 1 (1992): 1–22; Cueto, ed., *Missionaries of Science: The Rockefeller Foundation and Latin America* (Bloomington: Indiana University Press, 1994); Cueto, *The Value of Health: A History of the Pan American Health Organization* (Washington: Pan American Health Organization, 2007); Cueto, *Cold War, Deadly Fevers: Malaria Eradication in Mexico, 1955–1975* (Baltimore: Johns Hopkins University Press, 2007).

10. Louis Chevalier, *Le choléra, la première épidémie du XIXe siècle* (La Roche-sur-Yon: Imprimerie Centrale de l'Ouest, 1958); Asa Briggs, "Cholera and Society in the Nineteenth Century," *Past and Present* 19 (1961): 76–96; Richard J. Evans, "Epidemics and Revolutions: Cholera in Nineteenth-Century Europe," *Past and Present* 120 (1988): 123–46; Frank M. Snowden, "Cholera in Barletta 1910," *Past and Present* 132 (1991): 67–103; R. J. Morris, *Cholera 1832: The Social Response to an Epidemic* (New York: Holmes and Meier Publishers, 1976).

11. Jeffrey D. Needell, "The *Revolta Contra Vacina* of 1904: The Revolt against 'Modernization' in *Belle-Époque* Rio de Janeiro," *Hispanic American Historical Review* 67, no. 2 (1987): 233–69.

12. See Carrigan, "Privilege, Prejudice, and the Strangers' Disease in Nineteenth-Century New Orleans"; Carrigan, *The Saffron Scourge: A History of Yellow Fever in Louisiana, 1796–1905*. Whether people of African descent actually enjoyed a somewhat lesser susceptibility to yellow fever remains a matter of controversy. Some historians claim that it was this innate resistance to yellow fever that led plantation owners in the southern North American colonies and in the Caribbean to increasingly favor African slavery over other available forms of labor: Philip R. P. Coelho and Robert A. McGuire, "African and European Bound Labor in the British New World: The Biological

Consequences of Economic Choices," *Journal of Economic History* 57, no. 1 (1997): 83–115; Kenneth F. Kiple and Brian T. Higgins, "Yellow Fever and the Africanization of the Caribbean," in *Disease and Demography in the Americas,* ed. John W. Verano and Douglas H. Ubelaker (Washington: Smithsonian Institution Press, 1992). Others disagree, concluding that the argument grants too much credence to the racist claims of slaveowners: Sheldon J. Watts, "Yellow Fever Immunities in West Africa and the Americas in the Age of Slavery and Beyond: A Reappraisal," *Journal of Social History* 34, no. 4 (2001): 955.

13. Roderick E. McGrew, *Russia and the Cholera, 1823–1832* (Madison: University of Wisconsin Press, 1965), 11.

14. Briggs, "Cholera and Society in the Nineteenth Century," 80–81.

15. David Arnold, "Cholera and Colonialism in British India," *Past and Present* 113 (1986): 119.

16. Patricia M. E. Lorcin, "Imperialism, Colonial Identity, and Race in Algeria, 1830–1870: The Role of the French Medical Corps," *Isis* 90, no. 4 (1999): 661.

17. Myron Echenberg, *Black Death, White Medicine: Bubonic Plague and the Politics of Public Health in Colonial Senegal, 1914–1945* (Portsmouth, NH: Heinemann, 2002); Maryinez Lyons, "Sleeping Sickness, Colonial Medicine and Imperialism: Some Connections in the Belgian Congo," in *Disease, Medicine, and Empire: Perspectives on Western Medicine and the Experience of European Expansion,* ed. Roy MacLeod and Milton Lewis (New York: Routledge, 1988); Raymond E. Dumett, "The Campaign against Malaria and the Expansion of Scientific Medical and Sanitary Services in British West Africa, 1898–1910," *African Historical Studies* 1, no. 2 (1968) : 153–97.

18. Benjamin, *The United States and Cuba: Hegemony and Dependent Development, 1880–1934;* Susan J. Fernández, *Encumbered Cuba: Capital Markets and Revolt, 1878–1895* (Gainesville: University Press of Florida, 2002); Foner, *The Spanish-Cuban-American War and the Birth of American Imperialism, 1895–1902;* Jorge Ibarra, "Los mecanismos económicos del capital financiero obstaculizan la formación de la burguesía doméstica cubana (1898–1930)," *ISLAS* 79 (1984) : 71; Ibarra, *Cuba: 1898–1921, partidos políticos y clases sociales* (Havana: Editorial de Ciencias Sociales, 1992); Ibarra, *Prologue to Revolution: Cuba, 1898–1958,* trans. Marjorie Moore (Boulder: Lynne Rienner Publishers, 1998); Ibarra, *Máximo Gómez frente al imperio, 1898–1905* (Havana: Editorial de Ciencias Sociales, 2000); Francisco López Segrera, *Cuba: Capitalismo dependiente y subdesarrollo (1510–1959)* (Havana: Casa de las Américas, 1972); López Segrera, *Sociología de la colonia y neocolonia cubana, 1510–1959* (Havana: Editorial de Ciencias Sociales, 1989); López Segrera, *Cuba, cultura y sociedad (1510–1985)* (Havana: Editorial Letras Cubanas, 1989); Louis A. Pérez, Jr., *Cuba between Empires, 1878–1902* (Pittsburgh: University of Pittsburgh Press, 1983); Pérez, *Cuba under the Platt Amendment, 1902–1934* (Pittsburgh: University of Pittsburgh Press, 1986); Pérez, *Cuba and the United States: Ties of Singular Intimacy;* Pérez, *Cuba: Between Reform and Revolution,* 2nd ed. (Oxford: Oxford University Press, 1995). This is part of a larger scholarship on U.S.–Latin American relations, where U.S. domination of Latin American countries is seen through an explicitly imperial lens. See, for

example, Gilbert M. Joseph, Catherine C. Legrand, and Ricardo D. Salvatore, eds., *Close Encounters of Empire: Writing the Cultural History of U.S.–Latin American Relations* (Durham: Duke University Press, 1998); Lars Schoultz, *Beneath the United States: A History of U.S. Policy toward Latin America* (Cambridge: Harvard University Press, 1998).

19. Lyons, "Sleeping Sickness, Colonial Medicine and Imperialism: Some Connections in the Belgian Congo," 247; Michael Worboys, "Manson, Ross and Colonial Medical Policy: Tropical Medicine in London and Liverpool, 1899–1914," in *Disease, Medicine, and Empire: Perspectives on Western Medicine and the Experience of European Expansion,* ed. MacLeod and Lewis.

20. Maryinez Lyons, *The Colonial Disease: A Social History of Sleeping Sickness in Northern Zaire, 1900–1940* (Cambridge: Cambridge University Press, 1992).

21. Philip D. Curtin, *Death by Migration: Europe's Encounter with the Tropical World in the Nineteenth Century* (Cambridge: Cambridge University Press, 1989); Daniel R. Headrick, *The Tools of Empire: Technology and European Imperialism in the Nineteenth Century* (Oxford: Oxford University Press, 1981).

22. David Patrick Geggus, *Slavery, War, and Revolution: The British Occupation of Saint Domingue, 1793–1798* (Oxford: Claredon Press, 1982), 354–64; Michael Duffy, *Soldiers, Sugar, and Seapower: The British Expeditions to the West Indies and the War against Revolutionary France* (Oxford: Oxford University Press, 1987), 326–67.

23. Lyons, *The Colonial Disease: A Social History of Sleeping Sickness in Northern Zaire, 1900–1940.*

24. Florence Bretelle-Establet, "Resistance and Receptivity: French Colonial Medicine in Southwest China, 1898–1930," *Modern China* 25, no. 2 (1999): 173.

25. Frantz Fanon, *A Study in Dying Colonialism,* trans. Haakon Chevalier (New York: Grove Press, 1965), 122–23.

26. For example, Mark Harrison, *Public Health in British India: Anglo-Indian Preventive Medicine, 1859–1914* (Cambridge: Cambridge University Press, 1994).

CHAPTER 2

1. "Declared Yellow Fever," *New Orleans Daily Picayune,* September 7, 1897, 1–2.

2. "Uncle Sam's Boys Abandon Jackson Barracks Because of Fever Scare," *New Orleans Daily Picayune,* September 14, 1897, 1; "Soldiers Were the First to Flee: Regiment of United States Artillery Comes Here Today," *Atlanta Constitution,* September 14, 1897, 1; "Refugees Flock Here for Safety: Trains from Infected Districts Are Crowded with Them," *Atlanta Constitution,* September 16, 1897, 5.

3. "As Trainmen See It: The Great Fear Draws a Dead Line Three Hundred Miles from Here," *New Orleans Daily Picayune,* September 15, 1897, 7.

4. "Mint in New Orleans Shut Off: Government Unable to Ship Coin Wanted Elsewhere," *New York Times,* September 16, 1897, 1.

5. "The Torch Applied as a Result of the Terror among the People," *New Orleans Daily Picayune,* September 24, 1897, 1–2. See also "The Mayor Stands Firm," *New Orleans Daily Picayune,* September 25, 1897, 1–2.

6. "Quarantine's Farewell: The Frosts Everywhere Remove All Cause for Fear," *New Orleans Daily Picayune,* November 5, 1897, 1.

7. "Local Gossip of the Fever: A Great Many Families Get out of Town," *Jackson Daily Clarion-Ledger,* September 14, 1897, 1; "To the Citizens of Jackssn [sic]," *Jackson Daily Clarion-Ledger,* September 15, 1897, 8; "Around and about Town: Many More People Are Leaving the City," *Jackson Daily Bulletin,* September 16, 1897, 1; "Jackson Gets a Swift Shake: Population of Mississippi's Capital Has Stampeded," *Atlanta Constitution,* September 16, 1897, 1. The *Jackson Daily Bulletin,* a two-page, three-column newspaper, was started on September 16 by "several of the can't-get-away Clarion-Ledger printers . . . for the purpose of publishing reliable daily bulletins of the yellow-fever situation." For the next six weeks, it reported the telegraphic news of the progress of the yellow fever patients in Edwards, including who had had episodes of black vomit; which residents had upcoming shifts on the quarantine guard and the curfew patrol; and the fishing exploits and occasional horse races of Jackson's idled citizens.

8. "Around and about Town: Many More People Are Leaving the City," *Jackson Daily Bulletin,* September 16, 1897, 1.

9. Jackson's mayor, Ramsey Wharton, assured the public of his confidence that "none of our citizens were engaged in any such lawlessness" and that the culprits, if ever identified, would swiftly be brought to justice; "Mayor's Proclamation," *Jackson Daily Bulletin,* September 18, 1897, 1. No arrests, however, were ever reported.

10. "Quarantine Established," *Houston Daily Post,* September 7, 1897, 3.

11. "The Beaumont Death: People Are Scattering," *Galveston Daily News,* September 24, 1897, 1.

12. "Houston Trains Off," *Galveston Daily News,* September 28, 1897, 1.

13. "Train Held up at Rayne, LA: The Special with the Louisiana Doctors Not Allowed to Pass the Town," *Galveston Daily News,* September 30, 1897, 2. See also "Experience of Dr. Guiteras: Never Saw More Fright Than in Rural Sections of Louisiana," *Galveston Daily News,* October 1, 1897, 1.

14. "Steamship Lines Suspend," *Galveston Daily News,* October 12, 1897, 1; "Trade Paralyzed," *New York Herald,* October 12, 1897, 1.

15. "City's Gates Open to the Refugees: Atlanta Will Welcome All Who Come from Fever Districts," *Atlanta Constitution,* September 15, 1; "Refugees Reaching the City: One Hundred and Fifty Came in at 2 O'Clock This Morning," *Atlanta Constitution,* September 15, 1, "Refugees Flock Here for Safety: Trains from Infected Districts Are Crowded with Them," *Atlanta Constitution,* September 16, 1897, 5; "Will Inspect All Incoming Trains: Board of Health Holds Another Important Meeting," *Atlanta Constitution,* September 16, 1897, 5.

16. "City's Gates Open to Refugees: Atlanta Will Welcome All Who Come

from Fever Districts," *Atlanta Constitution,* September 15, 1897, 1; "Deca-
tur Won't Take Chances: Alabama Town Doubles Guard to Watch Incoming
Trains," *Atlanta Constitution,* September 15, 1897, 1; "Huntsville Is Ap-
prehensive: Rigid Quarantine Will Be Enforced by City Officials," *Atlanta
Constitution,* September 15, 1897, 1; "Montgomery Fears Atlanta: Alabama
Capital Quarantines the Georgia Statehouse Town," *Atlanta Constitution,*
September 15, 1897, 1; "Charleston Has Quarantined: Palmetto State's Me-
tropolis Guards against Yellow Fever," *Atlanta Constitution,* September 15,
1897, 1; "Augusta Closes Her Doors," *Atlanta Constitution,* September 16,
1897, 5; "Selma is Afraid of Atlanta: Declares Quarantine against the Gate
City," *Atlanta Constitution,* September 16, 1897, 5; "Will Shut Out Yellow
Jack: Wilmington, N.C. Quarantines," *Atlanta Constitution,* September 16,
1897, 5; "Welcomed by a Shotgun: The Treatment Atlantians Are Subjected to
in Charleston," *Atlanta Constitution,* September 27, 1897, 5.

17. "A Plea for Reason and Common Sense," *Atlanta Constitution,* September 29, 1897, 4.

18. "Stocks Were Heavy: Yellow Fever Affected Southern Roads, Whole
List Sympathized," *Atlanta Constitution,* September 17, 1897, 8.

19. "Three New Cases in Montgomery: The Citizens of the Alabama Capi-
tal Are Panic Stricken," *Atlanta Constitution,* October 20, 1897, 1. See also
"Once Hated Town Now Their Home: People of Montgomery Flee to This
City for Refuge," *Atlanta Constitution,* October 20, 1897, 3.

20. "Railroads Stop All Their Trains: Not a Wheel Moved Yesterday between Montgomery and Selma," *Atlanta Constitution,* October 19, 1897, 6.

21. Edmund Souchon, "True Origin of the Epidemic of Yellow Fever," *Journal of the American Medical Association* 35 (1900): 309.; J. H. White, "True
Origin of the Epidemic of 1897," New York, January 29, 1898, in United
States Marine-Hospital Service, *Annual Report of the Supervising Surgeon-
General of the Marine-Hospital Service of the United States for the Fiscal Year
1898* (Washington: Government Printing Office, 1899), 536–39. The yellow
fever outbreak in Ocean Springs was even noted in the Spanish press, although
the Cuban origin of the epidemic was not acknowledged; "El Vómito en los
Estados Unidos," *El Imparcial* (Madrid), September 9, 1897, 1.

22. Stanford E. Chaillé, "Report to the United States National Board
of Health on Yellow Fever in Havana and Cuba," in *Annual Report of the
National Board of Health, 1880,* ed. U.S. National Board of Health (Wash-
ington: Government Printing Office, 1881), 72–73; J. M. Woodworth, "A Brief
Review of the Organization and Purpose of the Yellow Fever Commission,"
*Public Health Reports and Papers Presented at the Meetings of the American
Public Health Association* 4 (1877–78). Two hundred million dollars was ap-
proximately 2.3% of the U.S. gross national product in 1878. See Nathan S.
Balke and Robert J. Gordon, "The Estimation of Prewar Gross National
Product: Methodology and New Evidence," *Journal of Political Economy* 97,
no. 1 (1989): 84. For more recent accounts of the events of 1878, see Kahled J.
Bloom, *The Mississippi Valley's Great Yellow Fever Epidemic of 1878* (Baton
Rouge: Louisiana State University Press, 1993); John H. Ellis, *Yellow Fever
and Public Health in the New South* (Lexington: University Press of Kentucky,

1992); Margaret Humphreys, *Yellow Fever and the South* (Baltimore: Johns Hopkins University Press, 1992).

23. "The Late Yellow Fever Epidemic," *New York Times,* November 30, 1878, 8. See also Ellis, *Yellow Fever and Public Health in the New South,* 38.

24. Chaillé, "Report to the United States National Board of Health on Yellow Fever in Havana and Cuba," 78.

25. Ibid., 67.

26. Dr. D. M. Burgess, U.S. sanitary and quarantine inspector to a U.S. Congressional committee, February 12, 1879, quoted in ibid., 102.

27. Ibid., 107.

28. Ibid.

29. Ibid., 83–84.

30. Ibid., 181.

31. The U.S. Marine Hospital Service, a division of the Department of the Treasury, was founded in 1798 to provide health care to sailors who fell ill while far from their homes. On the role of the USMHS in the development of southern quarantine measures in the 1880s, see Humphreys, *Yellow Fever and the South,* 113–30.

32. Wolfred Nelson, "Cuba in Its Relation to the Southern United States; Its Danger as a Disease-Producing and Distributing Center," in *Tenth Biennial Report of the State Board of Health of California for the Fiscal Years from June 30, 1886, to June 30, 1888* (Sacramento: California State Board of Health, 1888).

33. Humphreys, *Yellow Fever and the South,* 120–24.

34. George Sternberg, *Report on the Etiology and Prevention of Yellow Fever* (Washington: Government Printing Office, 1890).

35. United States Congress, Senate, *Proceedings of the Cuba and Florida Immigration Investigation, the Senate Committee on Immigration, the Senate Committee on Epidemic Diseases, and the House Committee on Immigration and Naturalization, Acting Jointly through Subcommittees at Havana, Cuba, and at Key West, Fla., December 28 to 31, 1892,* 52nd Congress, 2nd Session, Report No. 1263, Ser. 3072 (Washington: Government Printing Office, 1893), I.

36. Ibid.

37. Ibid., I–II.

38. Ibid., II.

39. Ibid., III.

40. "Spanish Troops Ill in Cuba," *New York Times,* April 4, 1895, 5.

41. "Safeguards against Yellow Fever," *New York Times,* April 4, 1895, 16. See also *New York Times,* March 25, 1895, 5.

42. "Ridicule for Rebels," *New York Times,* May 22, 1895.

43. Ángel de Larra y Cerezo, *Datos para la historia de la campaña sanitaria en la Guerra de Cuba: Apuntes estadísticos relativos del año 1896* (Madrid: Imprenta de Ricardo Rojas, 1901), 37–38.

44. José A. Martínez-Fortún Foyo, "Historia de la medicina en Cuba (1840–1958)," *Cuadernos de la historia de la salud pública* 98, no. 1 (2005);

W. F. Brunner, "Morbidity and Mortality in the Spanish Army during the Calendar Year 1897," *Public Health Reports* 13, no. 17 (April 29, 1898): 409.

45. "Yellow Fever Threatened," *New York Times,* May 12, 1895, 1.

46. "Guards against Yellow Fever," *New York Times,* May 19, 1895, 16. See also "Precautions against a Yellow Fever Epidemic," *New York Daily Tribune,* May 19, 1895, 4.

47. Walter Wyman to the Secretary of the Treasury, June 8, 1895 in United States Marine-Hospital Service, *Annual Report of the Supervising Surgeon-General of the Marine-Hospital Service of the United States for the Fiscal Year 1895* (Washington: Government Printing Office, 1896), 344–45. Wyman's warnings were widely reported as the summer progressed. Examples include, *New York Times,* June 16, 1895, 5; "Tampa Free from Yellow Fever: Government Precautions Taken to Prevent the Plague Getting a Foothold," *Chicago Daily Tribune,* July 6, 1895, 4; and "An Insidious Enemy: Yellow Fever Is Playing Havoc in Cuba," *Los Angeles Times,* July 12, 1895, 2.

48. Walter Wyman to C. F. Shoemaker, Chief, Revenue Cutter Service, Treasury Department, June 17, 1895, in United States Marine-Hospital Service, *Annual Report of the Supervising Surgeon-General of the Marine-Hospital Service of the United States for the Fiscal Year 1895,* 345–46.

49. C. S. Hamlin, Assistant Secretary, Treasury Department to Commanding Officer Revenue Steamer McLane, July 24, 1895, in *Annual Report of the Supervising Surgeon-General of the Marine-Hospital Service of the United States for the Fiscal Year 1895,* 346–47.

50. The patrols paid particular attention to the state of Florida, which seemed to be the most likely landing point for the Cuban vessels, but also covered the rest of the Gulf and southern Atlantic states. For letters about patrolling Florida, see Walter Wyman to Treasury Department, June 17 and 21, 1897; W. B. Howell, Treasury Department to John W. Linck, Special Agent, June 25, 1897; and W. B. Howell, Treasury Department to Commanding Officer U.S.S. Forward, July 21, 1897; for other states see Walter Wyman to Treasury Department, June 22, 1897; all found in United States Marine-Hospital Service, *Annual Report of the Supervising Surgeon-General of the Marine-Hospital Service of the United States for the Fiscal Year 1897* (Washington: Government Printing Office, 1899), 430–32.

51. United States Marine-Hospital Service, *Annual Report of the Supervising Surgeon-General of the Marine-Hospital Service of the United States for the Fiscal Year 1895,* 384–439.

52. Ibid., 393–94.

53. Sanitary Inspector D. M. Burgess, Marine Hospital Service to Surgeon General, Marine Hospital Service, May 25, 1895, in *Annual Report of the Supervising Surgeon-General of the Marine-Hospital Service of the United States for the Fiscal Year 1895,* 398.

54. Ibid., 398–99.

55. Ibid., 397–98.

56. Ibid., 428.

57. Ibid., 396.

58. Walter Wyman to the Secretary of the Treasury, December 4, 1895 in United States Marine-Hospital Service, *Annual Report of the Supervising Surgeon-General of the Marine-Hospital Service of the United States for the Fiscal Year 1896* (Washington: Government Printing Office, 1896), 387.

59. Ibid.

60. Ibid., 389.

61. Richard Olney to Enrique Dupuy de Lôme, February 7, 1896, in *Annual Report of the Supervising Surgeon-General of the Marine-Hospital Service of the United States for the Fiscal Year 1896*, 391.

62. De Larra y Cerezo, *Datos para la historia de la campaña sanitaria en la Guerra de Cuba: Apuntes estadísticos relativos del año 1896*, 38.

63. "Yellow Fever Aids the Rebels," *New York Times*, June 6, 1896, 5.

64. See, for example, "Scourged by Disease," *New York Times*, July 21, 1896, 5; "Yellow Fever in Cuba," *New York Daily Tribune*, August 26, 1896, 1; and "Yellow Fever and Smallpox in Cuba," *New York Daily Tribune*, September 1, 1896, 2.

65. "Cuba Scourged by Yellow-Fever," *Chicago Daily Tribune*, October 12, 1896, 8; Burgess to Walter Wyman, September 15, 1896 in United States Marine-Hospital Service, *Annual Report of the Supervising Surgeon-General of the Marine-Hospital Service of the United States for the Fiscal Year 1896*, 392.

66. Burgess to Walter Wyman, October 17, 1896 in *Annual Report of the Supervising Surgeon-General of the Marine-Hospital Service of the United States for the Fiscal Year 1896*. Burgess's fears were reported in "Cuba Must Be Watched," *New York Times*, October 27, 1896, 5.

67. Martínez-Fortún Foyo, "Historia de la medicina en Cuba (1840–1958)"; Brunner, "Morbidity and Mortality in the Spanish Army during the Calendar Year 1897," 409–10; "Bad State of Havana Hospitals," *Chicago Daily Tribune*, December 18, 1896.

68. The resolution is reproduced in "Report of Surg. P. H. Bailhache upon the Meeting of the American Public Health Association, at Buffalo, N.Y., September 28, 1896," in United States Marine-Hospital Service, *Annual Report of the Supervising Surgeon-General of the Marine-Hospital Service of the United States for the Fiscal Year 1896*, 16–18.

69. "International Responsibility with Regard to Epidemic Diseases," address by Walter Wyman, Surgeon General, United States Marine Hospital Service at the Pan-American Medical Congress in the City of Mexico, November 17, 1896, in United States Marine-Hospital Service, *Annual Report of the Supervising Surgeon-General of the Marine-Hospital Service of the United States for the Fiscal Year 1897*, 220.

70. "Report of Vital Statistics of Havana, Year 1901," File 1901/275, Letters Received 1899–1902, Records of the Military Government of Cuba, Record Group 140, National Archives, College Park, MD (hereafter MGC/RG 140).

71. Gobierno Civil de Santa Clara, "Memoria del estado de la provincia y resumen de los trabajos realizados con observaciones e indicaciones sobre la marcha administrativa de la misma," File 1899/1339, Letters Received 1899–1902, MGC/ RG 140.

72. H. S. Caminero, Sanitary Inspector, USMHS, "A Report on Yellow Fever at Santiago de Cuba," June 1, 1897, in United States Marine-Hospital Service, *Annual Report of the Supervising Surgeon-General of the Marine-Hospital Service of the United States for the Fiscal Year 1897*, 473–75. See also the comments on the history of yellow fever in Santiago found in M. J. Rosenau, Passed Assistant Surgeon, USMHS, to Supervising Surgeon General, USMHS, May 8, 1899, enclosed in Herman B. Parker, Assistant Surgeon, USMHS, to the Military Governor of Cuba, November 15, 1899, File 1899/2594, Letters Received, 1899–1902, MGC/ RG 140.

73. "Statement of Deaths Caused by Yellow Fever in Cienfuegos," in José M. Frías, Mayor, Cienfuegos, letter, July 15, 1899, File 1899/4285, Letters Received, 1899–1902, MGC/ RG 140.

74. United States Marine-Hospital Service, *Annual Report of the Supervising Surgeon-General of the Marine-Hospital Service of the United States for the Fiscal Year 1895*, 376; United States Marine-Hospital Service, *Annual Report of the Supervising Surgeon-General of the Marine-Hospital Service of the United States for the Fiscal Year 1896*, 378; United States Marine-Hospital Service, *Annual Report of the Supervising Surgeon-General of the Marine-Hospital Service of the United States for the Fiscal Year 1897*, 428.

75. W. F. Brunner, "Sanitary Report from Habana," *Public Health Reports* 12, no. 34 (August 20, 1897): 82.

76. "Result of the Autopsy: Prof. Proctor Died of Yellow Fever," *New York Times*, September 17, 1888, 1; see also Jo Ann Carrigan, "Privilege, Prejudice, and the Strangers' Disease in Nineteenth-Century New Orleans," *Journal of Southern History* 36, no. 4 (1970): 574.

77. W. F. Brunner, "Sanitary Report from Habana," *Public Health Reports* 12, no. 39 (September 24, 1897): 1028.

78. De Larra y Cerezo, *Datos para la historia de la campaña sanitaria en la Guerra de Cuba: Apuntes estadísticos relativos del año 1896*, 41–43.

79. Brunner, "Morbidity and Mortality in the Spanish Army during the Calendar Year 1897," 441.

80. Ibid.

81. "Un Barco Cementerio," *El Imparcial* (Madrid), October 19, 1897, 1.

82. Souchon, "True Origin of the Epidemic of Yellow Fever," 309.

83. Surgeon General Walter Wyman, "Our Sanitary Obligations," March 22, 1900, cited in Souchon, 308. For further details on the 1897 epidemic in the U.S. South, see contemporary newspaper articles such as "Dr. Guiteras Reports," *New York Daily Tribune*, September 10, 1897, 7, and "The South and Its Invaders," *New York Daily Tribune*, September 11, 1897, 6. For a recent account of the 1897 yellow fever epidemic in the U.S. South, see Humphreys, *Yellow Fever and the South*.

84. "The Yellow Fever Outbreak," *New York Daily Tribune*, September 8, 1897, 6.

85. "A National Board of Health," *Atlanta Constitution*, September 24, 1897, 4.

86. Walter Wyman to the Secretary of the Treasury, Marine Hospital Service, August 30, 1897 in "Letters Addressed to the Secretary of the Treasury,

Recommending an Investigation by Officers of the Marine Hospital Service into the Cause of Yellow Fever, with Special Reference to the Reported Discovery of the Yellow Fever Germ by Professor Sanarelli," in United States Marine-Hospital Service, *Report of the Commission of Medical Officers Detailed by Authority of the President to Investigate the Cause of Yellow Fever* (Washington: Government Printing Office, 1899), 3.

87. Their laboratory was only completed in mid-January 1898. They were ordered to leave Havana in March. As yellow fever was not generally prevalent during the early months of each year, the doctors had very little material with which to work. Eugene Wasdin, "Preliminary Report of Medical Officers Detailed by Direction of the President as a Commission to Investigate in Habana the Cause of Yellow Fever," November 1, 1898, in United States Marine-Hospital Service, *Annual Report of the Supervising Surgeon-General of the Marine-Hospital Service of the United States for the Fiscal Year 1898*, 587.

88. Proposals to gain control of Cuba to eradicate yellow fever in Havana began to circulate in the aftermath of the 1878 epidemic. "Our Duty in Regard to Memphis," *Manufacturer and Builder* 2, no. 9 (1879).

89. "Annexation of Cuba," *Chicago Daily Tribune*, June 19, 1884, 11.

90. Editorial, *New York Times*, July 16, 1884, 4. See also "At Washington," *Chicago Daily Tribune*, July 15, 1884, 7.

91. Benjamin Lee, "Do the Sanitary Interests of the United States Demand the Annexation of Cuba?" *Public Health Papers and Reports* 15 (1889): 51. Others agreed. Unsuccessful in his presidential run in 1884, Blaine, who would become Secretary of State in 1889, remarked that "it would be cheaper for the United States to buy the island from Spain at almost any cost rather than it should be a constant menace to the health and prosperity of the Southern States." See "Shall the United States Buy Cuba?" *Chicago Daily Tribune*, February 12, 1889, 1.

92. *New York Journal*, April 7, 1896.

93. *New York Journal*, September 8, 1897.

94. "As to Yellow Fever," *Houston Daily Post*, September 7, 1897, 4.

95. Editorial, *Houston Daily Post*, October 13, 1897, 4.

96. "Where to Fumigate—Havana," *Atlanta Constitution*, October 26, 1897, 6.

97. "Will Ask Congress to Aid Cuba: Senator Call of Florida Will Push the Matter This Winter," *Chicago Daily Tribune*, September 14, 1895, 5. Call also made this argument on the open floor of the Senate, *Congressional Record*, 54th Cong., 1 Sess. 1896, 28: 1969. The congressional leadership, however, soon declared that any public discussion of U.S. interests in Cuba was unseemly and inappropriate while the Cuban people were suffering under Spanish tyranny, and proponents of intervention thereafter couched their arguments principally in humanitarian terms. *Congressional Record*, 54th Cong., 1st Sess., 1896, 28: 3575.

98. Stewart L. Woodford to Secretary of State John Sherman, September 13, 1897, October 4, 1897, and October 5, 1897 in United States Department of State, *Papers Relating to the Foreign Relations of the United States,*

with the Annual Message of the President Transmitted to Congress, December 5, 1898 (Washington: Government Printing Office, 1901), 562–65, 73–79.

99. Stewart L. Woodford to Secretary of State John Sherman, September 13, 1897 in ibid., 562. See also Stewart L. Woodford to Secretary of State John Sherman, October 4, 1897, and October 5, 1897, in United States Department of State, *Papers Relating to the Foreign Relations of the United States, with the Annual Message of the President Transmitted to Congress, December 5, 1898,* 576, 79.

100. Stewart L. Woodford to Secretary of State John Sherman, September 13, 1897 in United States Department of State, *Papers Relating to the Foreign Relations of the United States, with the Annual Message of the President Transmitted to Congress, December 5, 1898,* 565. See also Stewart L. Woodford to Secretary of State John Sherman, October 4, 1897, and October 5, 1897, in United States Department of State, *Papers Relating to the Foreign Relations of the United States, with the Annual Message of the President Transmitted to Congress, December 5, 1898,* 576, 79.

101. "Dr. Hamilton and Fever," *New York Times,* May 5, 1898, 12.

CHAPTER 3

1. Margaret Humphreys, *Yellow Fever and the South* (Baltimore: Johns Hopkins University Press, 1992), 24–25.

2. For a discussion of John Snow's hypothesis and how he reached his findings about cholera, see particularly chapter 10 of Peter Vinten-Johansen et al., *Cholera, Chloroform, and the Science of Medicine: A Life of John Snow* (Oxford: Oxford University Press, 2003), 254–82.

3. Stanford E. Chaillé, "Report to the United States National Board of Health on Yellow Fever in Havana and Cuba," in *Annual Report of the National Board of Health, 1880,* ed. U.S. National Board of Health (Washington: Government Printing Office, 1881), 165–66.

4. A Treaty of Peace between the United States and Spain, Senate Document No. 62, Part 1, U.S. Congress, 55th Cong., 3d Sess. (Washington: Government Printing Office, 1899).

5. Joint Resolution of Congress for the Recognition of the Independence of Cuba, April 20, 1898, Congressional Record, 55th Cong., 2d Sess., 1898, 31:3988. This declaration is known as the Teller Resolution.

6. Even in the occupation's earliest months, when establishing control over the island and overseeing the evacuation of the tens of thousands of Spanish troops from Cuba were the most immediate concerns of U.S. authorities, wide-ranging efforts against yellow fever were initiated. The return of thousands of U.S. soldiers from the island was, of course, also a source of concern for U.S. health officers. The U.S. Marine Hospital Service (USMHS) implemented a stringent quarantine inspection of vessels carrying returning army personnel to prevent the spread of yellow fever. As during the war, sick and wounded soldiers were to be transported only to northern ports. See Walter Wyman to L. J. Gage, August 5, 1898, in United States Marine-Hospital Service, *Annual Report of the Supervising Surgeon-General of the Marine-Hospital Service of*

the United States for the Fiscal Year 1898 (Washington: Government Printing Office, 1899), 688–89; and United States Marine-Hospital Service, *Annual Report of the Supervising Surgeon-General of the Marine-Hospital Service of the United States for the Fiscal Year 1899* (Washington: Government Printing Office, 1901), 620. The remains of U.S. Army personnel who had succumbed to yellow fever were considered an additional threat of contagion. Although the bodies of soldiers killed in battle were returned to the United States immediately to be buried with honors, those who had died from yellow fever were ordered held in Cuba until the winter months when transporting them was deemed safe. Wyman reported, "In a few instances these bodies were shipped to other places, the health officers and relatives being notified by telegram and prompt interment advised without opening the caskets. The transfer of these deceased heroes was viewed with apprehension by all sanitary authorities and required close surveillance to prevent possible risk"; ibid., 643.

7. "Final Report of Major H. F. Hodges, Chief Engineer, Department of Cuba," August 1, 1902, Reports of Officials of the Military Government, 1901–1902, Records of the Military Government of Cuba, Record Group 140, National Archives, College Park, MD (hereafter MGC/ RG 140).

8. *Reglamento de higiene para la ciudad de Puerto-Príncipe* (Puerto-Príncipe: Tipografía "La Verdad," 1899), 2.

9. M. C. Harper and J. C. Mehan, Superintendents of the Department of Street Cleaning, July 1, 1899 to June 30, 1900 in Leonard Wood, *Civil Report of Major General Leonard Wood, Military Governor of Cuba, (1900) for the Period from December 20th, 1899 to December 31st 1900,* 12 vols. (Washington: Government Printing Office, 1901).

10. "Report of Lieutenant W. J. Barden, Corps of Engineers, U.S.A., Chief Engineer, City of Havana," August 29, 1901, File 1901/1652, Letters Received 1899–1902, MGC/ RG 140.

11. When a current is passed through seawater, the concentration of free chlorine in the water increases, creating a mild disinfectant; W. M. Black, Chief Engineer, Division of Cuba, to the Adjutant General, Division of Cuba, July 30, 1900, File 1900/2538, Letters Received 1899–1902, MGC/ RG 140.

12. Walter Reed to Surgeon General, U.S. Army, April 20, 1900. File 1900/2538, Letters Received 1899–1902, MGC/ RG 140. This document also presents the results of Reed's extensive experimental research on the disinfecting qualities of electrozone.

13. W. J. Barden, Chief Engineer, City of Havana, to the Adjutant General, Department of Cuba, February 26, 1901, File 1901/1652, Letters Received 1899–1902, MGC/ RG 140. See also Major Walter Reed to Surgeon General, U.S. Army, April 20, 1900, File 1900/2538, Letters Received 1899–1902, MGC/ RG 140.

14. W. J. Barden, Chief Engineer, City of Havana, to the Adjutant General, Department of Cuba, February 26, 1901, File 1901/1652, Letters Received 1899–1902, MGC/ RG 140. The corrosive properties of electrozone made maintaining these carts difficult; the iron components of the wagons were continuously painted with hot tar as a protectant. "Report of the operations of

the Engineer Department for Havana January 1900," File 1900/1273. Letters Received 1899–1902, MGC/ RG 140.

15. Telegram from General Wilson to Adjutant General, Division of Cuba, November 15, 1899, File 1899/6533, Letters Received, 1899–1902, MGC/ RG 140.

16. "Report of Public Works, carried out under the directions of the Chief Engineer, Department of Havana and the Chief Engineer, Division of Cuba, from the date of the U.S. Military Occupation of Cuba, to April 30, 1900," File 1900/5695, Letters Received, 1899–1902, MGC/ RG 140.

17. "Report of Public Works, carried out under the directions of the Chief Engineer, Department of Havana and the Chief Engineer, Division of Cuba, from the date of the U.S. Military Occupation of Cuba, to April 30, 1900," File 1900/5695, Letters Received, 1899–1902, MGC/ RG 140. This process of renovation took place across the island. In Santiago, the "buildings over which the United States flag is hoisted have been put in the best possible repair." Leonard Wood, Department of Santiago to John R. Brooke, Military Governor of Cuba, January 26, 1899, File 1900/773, Letters Received, 1899–1902, MGC/ RG 140. Reports on the repair and sanitation of buildings in Santa Clara and Matanzas can be found in Letters reporting on the conditions in Santa Clara, and Matanzas, File 1900/3293, Letters Received, 1899–1902, MGC/ RG 140; and Gobierno Civil de Santa Clara, *Memorias del estado de la Provincia y resumen de los trabajos realizados con observaciones e indicaciones sobre la marcha administrativa de la misma* (Havana: Imprenta "El Fígaro," 1900), File 1900/1339, Letters Received, 1899–1902, MGC/ RG 140. See also Report dated July 7, 1899 by Major R. Echeverría, Brigade Surgeon, U.S. Volunteers on the sanitary conditions in various smaller towns, File 1899/4426, Letters Received, 1899–1902, MGC/ RG 140; and Report of Brigadier General James Wilson, Military Governor of the Department of Matanzas and Santa Clara, September 7, 1899, File 1899/2594, Letters Received, 1899–1902, MGC/ RG 140.

18. "Report of Public Works, carried out under the directions of the Chief Engineer, Department of Havana and the Chief Engineer, Division of Cuba, from the date of the U.S. Military Occupation of Cuba, to April 30, 1900," File 1900/5695, Letters Received, 1899–1902, MGC/ RG 140.

19. Leonard Wood to William McKinley, President of the United States, November 27, 1898, General Correspondence, 1825–1898, Leonard Wood Papers, Manuscript Division, Library of Congress, Washington, DC.

20. W. M. Beach, Chief Engineer, Department of Havana to Adjutant General, Department of Havana. August 15, 1899. File 1899/4249, Letters Received, 1899–1902, MGC/ RG 140.

21. Ibid.

22. B. J. Cromwell to John R. Brooke, August 15, 1899, File 1899/5210, Letters Received, 1899–1902, MGC/ RG 140.

23. William H. Carter to the Adjutant General, Division of Cuba, August 27, 1899, File 1899/5210, Letters Received, 1899–1902, MGC/ RG 140.

24. A. H. Weber to W. M. Black, Chief Engineer, Department of Havana,

August 28, 1899, File 1899/5210, Letters Received, 1899–1902, MGC/ RG 140.

25. Cromwell was not satisfied. He continued to report further developments in the dredging of the harbor, insisting that the process be halted due to the threat of yellow fever to his troops stationed nearby: "dredging was again commenced about eight P.M. last night and continued at intervals till after midnight, immediately in front of the Custom House passenger landing and this building. It was discontinued this morning and the dredger and scows were hauled off and are now lying at the buoy, partly filled with the foul silt dredged last night, exposed to the rays of the sun, the odor from which is driven through the Custom House passenger landing, this building, and the buildings in the immediate locality, thereby endangering the health of all the occupants, except immunes"; B. J. Cromwell to John R. Brooke, August 25, 1899, File 1899/5210, Letters Received, 1899–1902, MGC/ RG 140.

26. Walter Wyman to Quartermaster General, U.S. Army, July 7, 1899, File 1899/4584, Letters Received, 1899–1902, MGC/ RG 140.

27. Leonard Wood to Adjutant General, Division of Cuba, August 9, 1899, File 1899/4636, Letters Received, 1899–1902, MGC/ RG 140.

28. Aviso de Cuarentena, Júcaro and San Fernando Railroad, File 1899/6117, Letters Received, 1899–1902, MGC/ RG 140.

29. Henry R. Carter, Sanitary Inspector, USMHS to Major O'Reilly, Chief Surgeon of the Division of Cuba, July 3, 1899, File 1899/4369, Letters Received, 1899–1902, MGC/ RG 140.

30. The experience of one such ship is recounted in Moale, Commanding Officer, Nuevitas, to Adjutant General, Division of Cuba, November 11, 1899, File 1899/6497, Letters Received, 1899–1902, MGC/ RG 140.

31. A very detailed description of the occupation's disinfection of baggage was prepared in response to a petition by the British Consul on behalf of a woman whose clothes had been ruined by the process. The occupation rejected the petition on the grounds that disinfection was necessary to protect public health. Helen Cadelick to Lionel Carden, Esq., British Consul, May 9, 1901, and Edward Carpenter to Adjutant General, Department of Cuba, May 22, 1901, File 1901/2408, Letters Received, 1899–1902, MGC/ RG 140.

32. F. J. Ives to Adjutant General, Department of Matanzas and Santa Clara, July 18, 1899, File 1899/4834, Letters Received, 1899–1902, MGC/ RG 140.

33. Treasury Department Regulations "on baggage and personal effects from Cuban ports for ports in the United States," June 17, 1899, File 1899/4584, Letters Received, 1899–1902, MGC/ RG 140. A later reference to this regulation can be found in F. R. Trotter, Acting Chief Quarantine Officer, Havana, to E. H. Humphrey, Assistant Quartermaster in Havana, May 20, 1901, Letters Received, 1899–1902, MGC/ RG 140.

34. John G. Davis, "Statistics of Births, Marriages, Deaths, Immigration, and Yellow Fever from 1890–1899," File 1900/910, Letters Received, 1899–1902, MGC/ RG 140. Spanish records of yellow fever deaths in Havana going back to 1871 were deemed fairly reliable by the occupation government. William C. Gorgas, "Report of Vital Statistics of the City of Havana made to

Brigadier General Leonard Wood, Military Governor," File 1900/275, Miscellaneous Records of Various Agencies, 1899–1902, MGC/ RG 140.

35. Surgeon General, U.S. Army, to William C. Gorgas. December 21, 1898, General Correspondence and Other Papers I, October 1894 to August 1899, William C. Gorgas Papers.

36. William C. Gorgas to William Ludlow, November 7, 1900, General Correspondence and Other Papers I, October 1894 to August 1899, William C. Gorgas Papers. Examples of the procedure to be followed in reporting and investigating possible yellow fever cases can be found in William C. Gorgas, Chief Sanitary Officer of Havana to the Adjutant General, Division of Cuba on the case of Mr. Hayes and how to report a case of yellow fever, October 4, 1900, File 1900/5522, Letters Received, 1899–1902, MGC/ RG 140; Orestes Ferrera, Governor, Province of Santa Clara to General Wood, Military Governor of Cuba reporting the death of Sr. Manuel Fernández, October 4, 1900, Letters Received, 1899–1902, MGC/ RG 140; and Carlos J. Finlay, Chairman, Yellow Fever Commission of Havana to Assistant Adjutant General in Charge of Civil Affairs, Havana, reporting on the results of 10 examinations of suspected yellow fever cases, November 23, 1900, File 1900/3939, Letters Received, 1899–1902, MGC/ RG 140.

37. William C. Gorgas, Article sent to the *Medical Record,* August 17, 1901, Addresses, Articles, and Reports, 1901–12 and Undated, William C. Gorgas Papers. For example, when a doctor in Nuevitas, Puerto Príncipe, failed to report a case of yellow fever for four days, the commanding officer of Puerto Príncipe personally pursued the matter. Major Hatfield, Commanding Officer, Province of Puerto Príncipe to Adjutant General, Division of Cuba, April 20, 1900, File 1900/2359, Letters Received, 1899–1902, MGC/ RG 140.

38. Frank J. Ives, Surgeon, U.S.V. to the Adjutant General, Department of Matanzas and Santa Clara, December 30, 1899, File 1900/173, Letters Received, 1899–1902, MGC/ RG 140.

39. William C. Gorgas, Chief Sanitary Officer of Havana to the Assistant Adjutant General, Division of Cuba, June 8, 1900, File 1900/3204, Letters Received, 1899–1902, MGC/ RG 140.

40. As the 1900 yellow fever epidemic surged the USMHS became overwhelmed and preparations were made for a second disinfecting station to be used exclusively for the purpose for disinfecting the homes and property of yellow fever victims. Valery Havard, Chief Surgeon, Division of Cuba to the Adjutant General, Division of Cuba, September 6, 1900, File 1900/4784, Letters Received, 1899–1902, MGC/ RG 140.

41. William C. Gorgas, Chief Sanitary Officer of Havana to the Assistant Adjutant General, Division of Cuba, June 8, 1900, File 1900/3204, Letters Received, 1899–1902, MGC/ RG 140.

42. Fitzhugh Lee, Military Governor Department of Western Cuba, to Major H. L. Scott, Assistant Adjutant General, Division of Cuba, June 15–16, 1900, and endorsements, File 1900/500, Letters Received, 1899–1902, MGC/ RG 140.

43. William C. Gorgas, Chief Sanitary Officer, City of Havana, to H. L. Scott, Assistant Adjutant General, Division of Cuba, enclosing examples of

the 15 forms used in this process, August 27, 1900, File 1900/3755, Letters Received, 1899–1902, MGC/ RG 140. This procedure is also described in William C. Gorgas, Article sent to the *Medical Record*, August 17, 1901, Addresses, Articles, and Reports, 1901–12 and Undated, William C. Gorgas Papers.

44. H. M. Binkley, Division of Engineering Inspectors to M. A. W. Shockley, Assistant Surgeon, Office of Chief Sanitary Officer of Havana, December 4, 1900, File 1900/6304, Letters Received, 1899–1902, MGC/ RG 140.

45. William C. Gorgas, Chief Sanitary Officer of Havana to the Assistant Adjutant General, Division of Cuba, June 8, 1900, File 1900/3204, Letters Received, 1899–1902, MGC/ RG 140.

46. Charles Raynard to Leonard Wood, Military Governor of Cuba, June 11, 1900, and José Estraviz to E. St. J. Greble, Superintendent of Charities and Hospitals, Division of Cuba, June 12, 1900, File 1900/3185, Letters Received, 1899–1902, MGC/ RG 140.

47. William C. Gorgas, Article sent to the *Medical Record,* August 17, 1901, Addresses, Articles, and Reports, 1901–12 and Undated, William C. Gorgas Papers.

48. Summary of the claim by Mr. Sobrado to the City of Cárdenas for destruction of property, September 29, 1899, File 1899/6302, Letters Received, 1899–1902, MGC/ RG 140.

49. William C. Gorgas, Article sent to the *Medical Record,* August 17, 1901, Addresses, Articles, and Reports, 1901–12 and Undated, William C. Gorgas Papers. Sadly, the vast majority of these records were destroyed by the U.S. government in 1911 and 1913 to save the expense of storage. Margareth Jorgensen, *Preliminary Inventory of the Records of the Military Government of Cuba (Record Group 140)* (Washington: National Archives, 1962).

50. Robert McCleave, Disbursing Officer, Caibarién Barracks, Department of Matanzas and Santa Clara to W. J. Lutz, 2nd Infantry, Adjutant, Caibarién Barracks, Department of Matanzas and Santa Clara, Report about Remedios and Caibarién, June 30, 1900, File 1900/3293, Letters Received, 1899–1902, MGC/ RG 140.

51. William C. Gorgas, Chief Sanitary Officer of the City of Havana to the Adjutant General, Division of Cuba, November 8, 1900, File 1900/3714, Letters Received, 1899–1902, MGC/ RG 140.

52. A. N. Stark, Acting Chief Surgeon, Department of Havana and Pinar del Río in 3rd endorsement to letter from Diego Tamayo, Secretary of State and Government to Leonard Wood, Military Governor of Cuba, July 6, 1900, File 1900/3330, Letters Received, 1899–1902, MGC/ RG 140. The proprietors of these establishments pressed the government for compensation, but their claims were summarily rejected: "The action was necessary for the protection of human life, and to prevent the spread of an epidemic, and was the same as that taken in all countries under similar circumstances. Payment will not be made." In 2nd endorsement to Diego Tamayo, Secretary of State and Government to Leonard Wood, Military Governor of Cuba, November 13, 1900, File 1900/4778, Letters Received, 1899–1902, MGC/ RG 140.

53. An inspection of Quemados during the yellow fever epidemic of the

summer of 1900 led to the following report: "The saloon called 'La Gloria' on Real Street owned and kept by an American called George is still in operation; a man named Albert Highland, alias Boxer, and his wife reside on San Federico Street and being non-immunes should be moved; Real No. 2 is also open in violation of the law." A. N. Stark, Acting Chief Surgeon, to Orlando Ducker, Military Sanitary Officer, Quemados, June 26, 1900, Miscellaneous Records of Various Agencies, Department of Cuba, 1899–1902, MGC/ RG 140.

54. Chief Surgeon's Office, Department of the Province of Havana and Pinar del Rio to Major Orlando Ducker, Sanitary Officer, Quemados. June 25, 1900. Miscellaneous Records of Various Agencies, Department of Cuba, 1899–1902, MGC/ RG 140.

55. "Address delivered before the District of Columbia Medical Association, Washington, D.C." n.d. (1902–1904?), Addresses, Articles, and Reports, 1901–12 and Undated, William C. Gorgas Papers.

56. William C. Gorgas, Chief Sanitary Officer, City of Havana, to Adjutant General, Division of Cuba, October 9, 1900, File 1900/4782, Letters Received, 1899–1902, MGC/ RG 140. William C. Gorgas, Chief Sanitary Officer of Havana in 1st endorsement to H. L. Scott, Assistant Adjutant General, Division of Cuba to William C. Gorgas, Chief Sanitary Officer, City of Havana, July 21, 1900, July 23, 1900, File 1900/3755, Letters Received, 1899–1902, MGC/ RG 140.

57. William C. Gorgas, Chief Sanitary Officer of the City of Havana to the Adjutant General, Division of Cuba, November 8, 1900, File 1900/3714, Letters Received, 1899–1902, MGC/ RG 140.

58. William C. Gorgas, Chief Sanitary Officer of Havana in 1st endorsement to H. L. Scott, Assistant Adjutant General, Division of Cuba, to Major William C. Gorgas, Chief Sanitary Officer, City of Havana, July 21, 1900, July 23, 1900, File 1900/3755, Letters Received, 1899–1902, MGC/ RG 140. Others made the same observation: Brigadier General William Ludlow, governor of the Department of the Province of Havana argued, "The main fact relative to the yellow fever in 1898, is that for two years previous—being the period of the war—all immigration had practically ceased, and the remaining population, from prolonged residence or previous attack, was substantially immune." He went on to note that three-fourths of Havana's yellow fever cases in 1899 were Spanish immigrants. Brigadier General William Ludlow, Military Governor of Havana to the Adjutant General, Division of Cuba, January 28, 1900, File 1900/761, Letters Received, 1899–1902, MGC/ RG 140.

59. William C. Gorgas, Chief Sanitary Officer of the City of Havana, "Report of Vital Statistics of Havana for September 1900," October 1, 1900, File 1900/5513, Miscellaneous Records of Various Agencies, Department of Cuba, 1899–1902, MGC/ RG 140.

60. William C. Gorgas to Adjutant General, Division of Cuba, October 9, 1900, File 1900/4782, Letters Received, 1899–1902, MGC/ RG 140.

61. Valery Havard, Chief Surgeon of the Division of Cuba, William C. Gorgas, Chief Sanitary Officer of the City of Havana, A. H. Glennan, Chief Quarantine Officer for the Island of Cuba, USMHS, Agustín Varona, Vicente Benito Valdés, and T. C. Lyster, U.S. Army, to H. L. Scott, Adjutant General for

the Division of Cuba, September 17, 1900, File 1900/4782, Letters Received, 1899–1902, MGC/ RG 140.

62. "Civil Order No. 451," November 6, 1900, in Wood, *Civil Report of Major General Leonard Wood, Military Governor of Cuba, (1900) for the Period from December 20th, 1899 to December 31st 1900.* Comments on the efforts to prevent immigrants from going to Havana and taking them directly to the countryside can be found in "Preventing Yellow Fever: Immigrants Forbidden to Land at Havana," *New York News,* November 11, 1900; "Havana Fever Conditions: Steps Which May Eventually Stop Its Spread in the City," *Globe Democrat,* St. Louis, Missouri, November 7, 1900; "Heading Off Yellow Fever: Immigrants Forbidden to Land at Havana," *New York News,* November 10, 1900; and "Yellow Fever Precautions at Havana," *New York Times,* November 8, 1900; found in William C. Gorgas's scrapbook on yellow fever in Havana, Item 29, William C. Gorgas Papers.

63. S. L. Beckwith, "Subordinates Direct Cuban Affairs during Absence of the Generals," *Atlanta Constitution,* October 31, 1900, File 1900/5936, Letters Received, 1899–1902, MGC/ RG 140.

64. Valery Havard to the Adjutant General, Division of Cuba, September 18, 1900, File 1900/5576, Letters Received, 1899–1902, MGC/ RG 140. S. L. Beckwith also discussed this in the article published in *Atlanta Constitution.*

65. Order Number 390, Havana, September 28, 1900, File 1900/6751, Letters Received, 1899–1902, MGC/ RG 140.

66. E. Ruiz to Chief of the Military Health Department of Matanzas, September 29, 1900, File 1900/5075, Letters Received, 1899–1902, MGC/ RG 140.

67. A. H. Glennan, Surgeon, USMHS, Chief Quarantine Officer for Island of Cuba. October 11, 1900, Endorsement to E. Ruiz to Chief of the Military Health Department of Matanzas, September 29, 1900, File 1900/5075, Letters Received, 1899–1902, MGC/ RG 140.

68. William C. Gorgas, "Sanitary Conditions as Encountered in Cuba and Panama, and What Is Being Done to Render the Canal Zone Healthy," read before the 4th Pan American Medical Congress, Panama, January 3–6, 1905, printed in the *Medical Record,* February 4, 1905 (William Wood and Company, New York), Addresses, Articles-1905, William C. Gorgas Papers.

69. José Bubchura, Pedro Kade, and Azar T. Azar to John R. Brooke, Military Governor of Cuba, October 24, 1899; Domingo Méndez Capote, Secretary of State and Government, Pinar del Río to John R. Brooke, Military Governor of Cuba, October 25, 1899; Guillermo Dolz, Office of the Civil Governor of Pinar del Río to Quirico Callostra, Consul General of Turkey, October 25, 1899; and Guillermo Dolz, Office of the Civil Governor of Pinar del Río to the Secretary of State and Government in Havana, October 25, 1899, File 1899/6288, Letters Received, 1899–1902, MGC/ RG 140.

70. C. F. Carbonell to Major H. L. Scott, Adjutant General, Division of Cuba, October 6, 1900, and November 2, 1900, File 1900/5390, Letters Received, 1899–1902, MGC/ RG 140.

71. Noble David Cook, *Born to Die: Disease and New World Conquest, 1492–1650* (Cambridge: Cambridge University Press, 1998), 152–53.

72. Ramon Powers and James N. Lieker, "Cholera among the Plains Indians: Perceptions, Causes, Consequences," *Western Historical Quarterly* 29, no. 3 (1998): 338.

73. David Arnold, *Colonizing the Body: State Medicine and Epidemic Disease in Nineteenth-Century India* (Berkeley: University of California Press, 1993), 213. The pattern of infection also played a role in Indian resistance: few Europeans came down with the disease, raising suspicions that the plague was a British plot to kill unwanted Indians (Arnold, 208).

74. Florence Bretelle-Establet, "Resistance and Receptivity: French Colonial Medicine in Southwest China, 1898–1930," *Modern China* 25, no. 2 (1999): 171–203.

75. See, for example, Graham A. Cosmas, "Securing the Fruits of Victory: The U.S. Army Occupies Cuba, 1898–1899," *Military Affairs* 38, no. 3 (1974): 85–91; Vincent J. Cirillo, *Bullets and Bacilli: The Spanish-American War and Military Medicine* (New Bruswick: Rutgers University Press, 2004); John Lawrence Tone, *War and Genocide in Cuba, 1895–1898* (Chapel Hill: University of North Carolina Press, 2006).

76. L. G. Carr, Chief Surgeon, District of Santiago to the Adjutant General, District of Santiago, July 1, 1901, File 1901/3331, Letters Received, 1899–1902, MGC/ RG 140, and William C. Gorgas, "Report of Vital Statistics of Havana for the Year 1900," Miscellaneous Records of Various Agencies, Department of Cuba, 1899–1902, MGC/ RG 140.

77. William C. Gorgas, "Malaria in the Tropics," read at the Annual Meeting of the American Society of Tropical Medicine, Philadelphia, March 24, 1906, printed in the *Journal of the American Medical Association,* May 5, 1906, Addresses, Articles-1906–07, William C. Gorgas Papers.

78. Some examples are Robert E. Welch, Jr. , "William McKinley: Reluctant Warrior, Cautious Imperialist," in *Traditions and Values: American Diplomacy, 1865–1945,* ed. Norman A. Graebner (Lanham, MD: University Press of America, 1985); Albert Shaw, *International Bearings of American Policy* (Baltimore: Johns Hopkins University Press, 1943); James C. Bradford, "Introduction," in *Crucible of Empire: The Spanish-American War and Its Aftermath,* ed. James C. Bradford (Annapolis: Naval Institute Press, 1993).

79. James H. Hitchman, "Unfinished Business: Public Works in Cuba, 1898–1902," *The Americas* 31, no. 3 (1975): 337.

80. M. J. Rosenau, Passed Assistant Surgeon, USMHS to the Supervising Surgeon General, USMHS, "Mortuary Statistics from Santiago de Cuba," May 8, 1899, File 1899/2594, Letters Received, 1899–1902, MGC/ RG 140.

81. William C. Gorgas, *Report of Vital Statistics for the City of Havana for the Year 1900,* Miscellaneous Records of Various Agencies, 1899–1902, MGC/ RG 140.

82. Leonard Wood, Military Governor of Cuba to Elihu Root, Secretary of War, October 18, 1901, General Correspondence, 1901, Leonard Wood Papers.

83. William C. Gorgas, "Sanitary Conditions as Encountered in Cuba and Panama, and What Is Being Done to Render the Canal Zone Healthy," read before the 4th Pan American Medical Congress, Panama, January 3–6, 1905,

printed in the *Medical Record,* February 4, 1905, Addresses, Articles-1905, William C. Gorgas Papers.

84. William C. Gorgas, "Report of Vital Statistics of the City of Havana made to Brigadier General Leonard Wood, Military Governor," File 1900/275, Miscellaneous Records of Various Agencies, 1899–1902, MGC/ RG 140.

85. Dozens of such newspaper stories can be found in Gorgas's scrapbook on yellow fever in Havana, Item 29, William C. Gorgas Papers.

86. See, for example, "General Wood on Havana's Yellow Fever," *New York Sun,* November 8, 1900.

87. "Disappearance of Yellow Fever from Havana, Cuba," read before the Academy of Medicine, New York (1902–1904), Addresses, Articles, and Reports, 1901–12, and Undated, William C. Gorgas Papers.

88. B. E. Hambleton, Acting Collector, Office of the Collector of Customs, Port of Santiago to the Collector of Customs for the Island of Cuba, August 5, 1899; and Captain T. F. Davis, Collector of Customs, Port of Santiago to the Collector of Customs for the Island of Cuba, August 15, 1899, File 1899/5271, Letters Received, 1899–1902, MGC/ RG 140.

89. "Major Peterson's Fine Record," *New York Tribune,* October 18, 1900; and S. L. Beckwith, "Subordinates Direct Cuban Affairs during Absence of the Generals," *Atlanta Constitution,* October 31, 1900, File 1900/5936, Letters Received, 1899–1902, MGC/ RG 140.

90. "Disappearance of Yellow Fever from Havana, Cuba," read before the Academy of Medicine, New York, (1902–1904), Addresses, Articles, and Reports, 1901–12, and Undated, William C. Gorgas Papers. See also "Havana's Fever Scourge: Yellow Jack Has Been More Virulent Than Usual This Summer— Physicians Hard Pressed," *Brooklyn Eagle,* October 9, 1900, found in Gorgas's scrapbook on yellow fever in Havana, Item 29, William C. Gorgas Papers.

91. Leonard Wood to Adjutant General, Division of Cuba, August 9, 1899, File 1899/4636, Letters Received, 1899–1902, MGC/ RG 140.

92. Leonard Wood, Military Governor of Cuba to Elihu Root, Secretary of War, June 27, 1900, General Correspondence, 1899, Leonard Wood Papers.

CHAPTER 4

1. Nancy Stepan, "The Interplay between Socio-Economic Factors and Medical Science: Yellow Fever Research, Cuba and the United States," *Social Studies of Science* 8, no. 4 (1978) : 397–423; John Lawrence Tone, *War and Genocide in Cuba, 1895–1898* (Chapel Hill: University of North Carolina Press, 2006); Emilio Roig de Leuchsenring, *Médicos y medicina en Cuba* (Havana: Museo Histórico de las Ciencias Médicas "Carlos Finlay," 1965).

2. Howard A. Kelly, *Walter Reed and Yellow Fever* (New York: McClure, Phillips and Co., 1906); Albert E. Truby, *Memoir of Walter Reed: The Yellow Fever Episode* (New York: Paul B. Hoeber, 1943); Paul de Kruif, *Microbe Hunters* (New York: Harcourt, Brace, and Co., 1926); Sidney Howard and Paul de Kruif, *Yellow Jack: A History* (New York: Harcourt, Brace, and Co., 1933). This perspective is repeated in countless later works.

3. Stanford E. Chaillé, "Report to the United States National Board of Health on Yellow Fever in Havana and Cuba," in *Annual Report of the National Board of Health, 1880,* ed. U.S. National Board of Health (Washington: Government Printing Office, 1881), 67.

4. Carlos J. Finlay, "El mosquito hipotéticamente considerado como agente de transmisión de la fiebre amarilla," *Anales de la Academia de Ciencias Médicas, Físicas y Naturales de La Habana* 18 (1881): 147–69.

5. Some scholars have argued that Finlay's theory was merely one step beyond what others had been working on and that he purposely did not give credit to scientists such as Patrick Manson, who had already suggested that malaria was caused by a mosquito bite, Alphonse Laveran, who had posited that a malaria parasite must be found outside of the human body, and Ronald Ross, who proved Manson's theory. François Delaporte, *The History of Yellow Fever: An Essay on the Birth of Tropical Medicine,* trans. Arthur Goldhammer (Cambridge: MIT Press, 1991).

6. Finlay, "El mosquito hipotéticamente considerado como agente de transmisión de la fiebre amarilla."

7. For the explanation that Finlay was ignored because U.S. sanitarians believed Latin Americans to be inferior, see Stepan, "The Interplay between Socio-Economic Factors and Medical Science," 410. For an example of contemporary criticism of Finlay, see George H. F. Nuttall, "On the Role of Insects, Arachnids and Myriapods as Carriers in the Spread of Bacteria and Parasitic Diseases of Man and Animals: A Critical and Historical Study," *Johns Hopkins Reports* 8 (1899–1900): 1–152.

8. Margaret Humphreys, *Yellow Fever and the South* (Baltimore: Johns Hopkins University Press, 1992), 36–37; Stepan, "The Interplay between Socio-Economic Factors and Medical Science," 410.

9. Walter Reed et al., "The Etiology of Yellow Fever—A Preliminary Note," in *Yellow Fever: A Compilation of Various Publications,* ed. U.S. Senate (Washington: Government Printing Office, 1911 [1900]), 57, 59.

10. Jesse W. Lazear to Mabel H. Lazear, July 15, 1900, File 00334001, Jesse Lazear Series, Philip S. Hench Walter Reed Yellow Fever Collection, the Claude Moore Health Sciences Library, University of Virginia, Charlottesville, VA.

11. Walter Reed, "The Propagation of Yellow Fever—Observations Based on Recent Researches," in *Yellow Fever: A Compilation of Various Publications,* ed. U.S. Senate (Washington: Government Printing Office, 1911 [1901]), 94; Kelly, *Walter Reed and Yellow Fever,* 127; Truby, *Memoir of Walter Reed: The Yellow Fever Episode,* 89.

12. Henry R. Carter, "A Note on the Interval between Infecting and Secondary Cases of Yellow Fever from the Records of the Yellow Fever at Orwood and Taylor, Miss., in 1898," *New Orleans Medical and Surgical Journal* 52, no. 11 (1900): 618–36.

13. Henry R. Carter to Jesse Lazear, June 26, 1900, Henry Rose Carter Papers, Manuscript Collection 160, History of Medicine Division, National Library of Medicine, Bethesda, MD. Transcription and photograph of note also appear in Ralph Chester Williams, *The United States Public Health Service,*

1798–1950 (Washington: Commissioned Officers Association of the United States Public Health Service, 1951), 260.

14. Reed et al., "The Etiology of Yellow Fever—A Preliminary Note," 62.

15. Walter Reed to Emily Lawrence Reed, August 2, 1900, Walter Reed Series, File 02077001, Philip S. Hench Walter Reed Yellow Fever Collection, the Claude Moore Health Sciences Library, University of Virginia, Charlottesville, VA.

16. Jesse W. Lazear to Mabel H. Lazear, August 23, 1900, File 00341001, Jesse Lazear Series, Philip S. Hench Walter Reed Yellow Fever Collection.

17. Reed et al., "The Etiology of Yellow Fever—A Preliminary Note," 63.

18. Walter Reed to James Carroll, September 7, 1900, File 15312004, James Carroll Papers, Edward Hook Additions to the Philip S. Hench Walter Reed Yellow Fever Collection, the Claude Moore Health Sciences Library, University of Virginia, Charlottesville, VA.

19. Reed et al., "The Etiology of Yellow Fever—A Preliminary Note," 66–67.

20. Jefferson R. Kean to Mabel H. Lazear, September 26, 1900, File 00358001, Jesse Lazear Series, Philip S. Hench Walter Reed Yellow Fever Collection.

21. Reed et al., "The Etiology of Yellow Fever—A Preliminary Note," 68–69.

22. Walter Reed to James Carroll, September 24, 1900, File 02124001, Walter Reed Series, Philip S. Hench Walter Reed Yellow Fever Collection.

23. Walter Reed to Emilie Lawrence Reed, October 6, 1900, File 02135001, Walter Reed Series, Philip S. Hench Walter Reed Yellow Fever Collection.

24. Jefferson R. Kean to Hagedorn, June 12, 1929, File 06283006, Jefferson Randolph Kean Series, Philip S. Hench Walter Reed Yellow Fever Collection, the Claude Moore Health Sciences Library, University of Virginia, Charlottesville, VA.

25. Some have argued that Reed moved quickly to present the findings because of the presence of two British scientists on the island who allegedly "helped" Reed make the connection between the intrinsic incubation period proposed by Carter and the disease. See Delaporte, *The History of Yellow Fever: An Essay on the Birth of Tropical Medicine*. The documents reveal that is not the case.

26. Walter Reed, James Carroll, and Arístides Agramonte, "The Etiology of Yellow Fever—An Additional Note," in *Yellow Fever: A Compilation of Various Publications,* ed. U.S. Senate (Washington: Government Printing Office, 1911 [1901]), 70.

27. Ibid., 74–81.

28. "¡Horrendo . . . si es cierto!: ¡La fiebre amarilla inoculada a los inmigrantes españoles por medio de mosquitos!" *La Discusión,* November 21, 1900. Upset by the rumors, Reed asked the Spanish consul to make a statement. Walter Reed to Emilie Lawrence Reed, November 22, 1900, File 02213001, Walter Reed Series, Philip S. Hench Walter Reed Yellow Fever Collection. The reassurances of the Spanish consul that some of the volunteers were from the

United States and that the Spanish immigrants had knowingly agreed to participate appeared on the front page of *La Discusión* two days later. "La Fiebre amarilla: inoculación por los mosquitos—entrevista con el cónsul español," *La Discusión,* November 24, 1900.

29. Reed, Carroll, and Agramonte, "The Etiology of Yellow Fever—An Additional Note," 74–75.

30. Informed Consent Agreement for Antonio Benigno, November 26, 1900, File 07003001, Diplomas and Certificates, Philip S. Hench Walter Reed Yellow Fever Collection, the Claude Moore Health Sciences Library, University of Virginia, Charlottesville, VA.

31. Ibid.

32. William C. Gorgas, *Sanitation in Panama* (New York: D. Appleton and Co., 1915), 25.

33. Ibid., 30–31.

34. Reed, Carroll, and Agramonte, "The Etiology of Yellow Fever—An Additional Note," 84. "Infected (soiled) bedding and clothing at Camp Lazear, near Buena Vista, Cuba, December 20, 1900," File KAMD0310, the Jefferson Randolph Kean Paper, Philip S. Hench Walter Reed Yellow Fever Collection.

35. Reed, Carroll, and Agramonte, "The Etiology of Yellow Fever—An Additional Note," 87.

36. William C. Gorgas to Henry R. Carter, December 13, 1900, File 02237001, Walter Reed Series, Philip S. Hench Walter Reed Yellow Fever Collection. As it turned out, Carter was not able to rejoin Gorgas for the "historic campaign" against yellow fever in Havana. Gorgas did successfully recruit Carter for his next battle against the disease, however, in the Panama Canal Zone beginning in 1904, and the two friends continued to work closely together frequently in the fight against yellow fever until Gorgas's death in 1920.

37. This is not to suggest that basic sanitation was neglected. In July 1901 Gorgas commented: "I think that we should not relax any effort that tends in the direction of improving the hygiene of the city." Gorgas to the Adjutant General, July 24, 1901, File 1901/71, Letters Received, 1899–1902, Records of the Military Government of Cuba, Record Group 140, National Archives, College Park, MD (hereafter MGC/ RG 140.) Some previously lauded measures, however, were discredited. The general use of electrozone, for example, was discontinued in February 1901; "In the light of our recently acquired knowledge concerning the transmission of yellow fever and malaria by the mosquito, the usefulness of electrozone, except as a deodorant, is to say the least problematic, and I would recommend that its manufacture be discontinued." Valery Havard, Endorsements to letter of Henry G. Piffard to Governor Wood, February 7, 1901, File 1901/1005, Letters Received, 1899–1902, MGC/ RG 140. Indeed, Gorgas discouraged others from building electrozone plants. William C. Gorgas to Dr. Woodbury, Commissioner of Street Cleaning of New York City, March 29, 1902, General Correspondences and other papers-I, 1894, October–1899, August, William C. Gorgas Papers, Manuscript Division, Library of Congress, Washington, DC.

38. J. A. López to William C. Gorgas, July 2, 1901, General Correspon-

dence and other papers-I, 1894, October–1899, August, William C. Gorgas Papers. A third Special Disinfection Brigade was tasked with cases of all other infectious diseases.

39. William C. Gorgas to the Adjutant General, August 30, 1901, Semi-annual report of the Sanitary Department–six months ending June 30, 1901, File 1901/2859, Letters Received, 1899–1902, MGC/ RG 140.

40. The fumes of sulfur and tobacco kill mosquitoes outright, which made these substances easier to use than pyrethrum, but they also damage fabrics, which led the authorities to consider them unsuitable for general use. William C. Gorgas, Assistant Surgeon General, "Address delivered before the District of Columbia Medical Association, Washington, D.C." n.d. (1902–1904), Addresses, Articles, and Reports, 1901–12 and Undated, William C. Gorgas Papers.

41. Draft of Report of Brigadier General Leonard Wood, File 1, Reports of Officials of the Military Government, 1901–1902, MGC/ RG 140.

42. "Report of Vital Statistics of Havana, Guanabacoa, and Regla, April 1901," William C. Gorgas Papers.

43. Ibid.

44. William C. Gorgas to the Adjutant General, August 30, 1901, Semi-annual report of the Sanitary Department–six months ending June 30, 1901, File 1901/2859, Letters Received, 1899–1902, MGC/ RG 140.

45. Miguel Gener, Municipal Alcalde of Havana, Order of May 6, 1901, General Correspondence and other papers-I, 1894, October–1899, August, William C. Gorgas Papers.

46. Joseph A. Le Prince, Assistant to Chief Sanitary Officer, to William C. Gorgas, Chief Sanitary Officer of Havana, May 19, 1902, File 2, Reports of Officials of the Military Government, 1901–1902, MGC/ RG 140.

47. William C. Gorgas to the Adjutant General, August 30, 1901, Semi-annual report of the Sanitary Department–six months ending June 30, 1901, File 1901/2859, Letters Received, 1899–1902, MGC/ RG 140.

48. William C. Gorgas, Chief Sanitary Officer, to Brigadier General Leonard Wood, "Report of Vital Statistics of the City of Havana, Year 1901," Miscellaneous Records of Various Agencies, Department of Cuba, 1899–1902, MGC/ RG 140.

49. Those who complained usually blamed their neighbors' failures to take adequate measures against mosquitoes, "but in nearly every case we have found the mosquitoes to be breeding on their premesis [sic]." Joseph A. Le Prince, Assistant to Chief Sanitary Officer, to William C. Gorgas, Chief Sanitary Officer of Havana, May 19, 1902, File 4, Reports of Officials of the Military Government, 1901–1902, MGC/ RG 140.

50. "Report of Vital Statistics of Havana, Guanabacoa, and Regla, March 1901," File 1901/275, Letters Received, 1899–1902, MGC/ RG 140.

51. Joseph A. Le Prince, Assistant to Chief Sanitary Officer, to William C. Gorgas, Chief Sanitary Officer of Havana, May 19, 1902, File 4, Reports of Officials of the Military Government, 1901–1902, MGC/ RG 140.

52. R. Galbis to Leonard Wood, July 17, 1901, File 1901/3214, Letters Received, 1899–1902, MGC/ RG 140.

53. Rita López to Leonard Wood, n.d., File 1901/578, Letters Received, 1899–1902, MGC/ RG 140.

54. William C. Gorgas to the Adjutant General, June 2, 1901 and Order No. 157, Headquarters Department of Cuba, Havana, June 12, 1901, File 1901/2774, Letters Received, 1899–1902, MGC/ RG 140.

55. L. G. Carr, Chief Surgeon, District of Santiago to Adjutant General, District of Santiago, July 1, 1901, File 1901/3331, Letters Received, 1899–1902, MGC/ RG 140.

56. D. Lombillo Clark, "Informes relativos a las obras y servicios que corrían a cargo de los Ingenieros Militares entregados por éstos al Departamento antes del 19 de mayo de 1902," Reports of Officials of the Military Government, 1901–1902, MGC/ RG 140.

57. Hamilton Stone to the Adjutant, Hamilton Barracks, Cuba, October 12, 1901 and letter endorsements, File 1901/2696, Letters Received, MGC/ RG 140.

58. F. E. Trotter, Assistant Surgeon, U.S. Marine Hospital Service to 2nd Lt. E. H. Humphreys, Acting Assistant Quartermaster in Havana, May 20, 1901, File 1901/1401, Letters Received, 1899–1902, MGC/ RG 140; Resolution of the Louisiana State Board of Health, June 3, 1901, File 1901/1401, Letters Received, 1899–1902, MGC/ RG 140.

59. "Report of Vital Statistics of Havana, Guanabacoa, and Regla, March 1901," File 1901/275, Letters Received, 1899–1902, MGC/ RG 140.

60. "Report of Vital Statistics of Havana, Guanabacoa, and Regla, April 1901," William C. Gorgas Papers.

61. "Report of Vital Statistics of Havana, Guanabacoa, and Regla, June 1901," File 1901/275, Letters Received, 1899–1902, MGC/ RG 140.

62. "Report of Vital Statistics of Havana, Guanabacoa, and Regla, July 1901," File 1901/275, Letters Received, 1899–1902, MGC/ RG 140.

63. "Report of Vital Statistics of Havana, Guanabacoa, and Regla, August 1901," File 1901/275, Letters Received, 1899–1902, MGC/ RG 140.

64. Henry Noyes, Commanding Officer, Hamilton Barracks, Matanzas, to the Adjutant General, Department of Cuba, July 1, 1901, File 1901/3331, Letters Received, 1899–1902, MGC/ RG 140.

65. Samuel M. Whiteside, Commanding Officer, District of Santiago to the Adjutant General, Department of Cuba, July 1, 1901, File 1901/3331, Letters Received, 1899–1902, MGC/ RG 140.

66. William C. Gorgas to Henry R. Carter, October 8, 1901, General Correspondence and other papers I, 1894, October–1899, August, William C. Gorgas Papers.

67. Henry R. Carter to William C. Gorgas, July 21, 1901, General Correspondence and other papers-I, 1894, October-1899, August, William C. Gorgas Papers.

68. Joaquín Jacobsen and J. Santos Fernández, Academy of Sciences of Havana, to the Military Governor of the Island of Cuba, March 13, 1902, File 1902/224, Letters Received, 1899–1902, MGC/ RG 140.

69. William C. Gorgas, *Report of Vital Statistics of the City of Havana, Year 1901*, File 1900/275, Letters Received, 1899–1902, MGC/ RG140.

70. William C. Gorgas, Chief Sanitary Officer of Havana, to J. Santos Fernández and Joaquín Jacobsen, April 21, 1902, File 1902/224, Letters Received, 1899–1902, MGC/ RG 140.

71. Samuel M. Whiteside, Commanding Officer, District of Santiago, to Adjutant General of Cuba, January 30, 1902, File 1901/3331, Letters Received, 1899–1902, MGC/ RG 140.

72. William C. Gorgas, "Semi-Annual Report of the Sanitary Department of Havana," August 30, 1901, File 1901/2859, Letters Received, 1899–1902, MGC/ RG 140.

73. William C. Gorgas, *Report of Vital Statistics of the Cities of Havana and Guanabacoa, January 1902,* February 18, 1902, File 1900/275, Letters Received, 1899–1902, MGC/ RG 140.

74. William C. Gorgas, *Report of Vital Statistics of the Cities of Havana and Guanabacoa, April 1902,* May 9, 1902, File 1900/275, Letters Received 1899–1902, MGC/ RG 140.

75. William C. Gorgas, Chief Sanitary Officer of the City of Havana, "Report of Vital Statistics of Havana for May 1902," July 12, 1902, Reports of Officials of the Military Government, 1901–1902, MGC/ RG 140.

76. Leonard Wood, *Civil Report of Brigadier General Leonard Wood, Military Governor of Cuba (1902)* (Washington: Government Printing Office, 1902), 196.

77. Gregorio M. Guiteras, "Report of the Epidemic of Yellow Fever of 1903 at Laredo, Minera, and Canal, Tex.," in United States Public Health and Marine-Hospital Service, *Annual Report of the Surgeon-General of the Public Health and Marine-Hospital Service of the United States for the Fiscal Year 1903* (Washington: Government Printing Office, 1904), 303–25.

78. William C. Gorgas to Secretary of War, "Sanitation of Guayaquil," January 9, 1913, Yellow Fever—Miscellaneous Papers, William C. Gorgas Papers.

79. Joseph Porter, State Health Officer of Florida, to William C. Gorgas, July 15, 1902, General Correspondence and other papers-I, 1902, May–August 27, William C. Gorgas Papers.

CHAPTER 5

1. For examples of the extensive historiography examining other aspects of the Platt Amendment see Lejeune Cummins, "The Formulation of the Platt Amendment," *The Americas* 23, no. 4 (1967): 370–88; James H. Hitchman, "The Platt Amendment Revisited: A Bibliographical Survey," *The Americas* 23, no. 4 (1967): 343–69; Jorge Ibarra, *Cuba: 1898–1921, partidos políticos y clases sociales* (Havana: Editorial de Ciencias Sociales, 1992); Luis Machado y Ortega, *La Enmienda Platt* (Havana: Imprenta "El Siglo XX," 1922); Manuel Márquez Sterling, *Proceso histórico de la Enmienda Platt (1897–1934)* (Havana: Imprenta "El Siglo XX," 1941); Louis A. Pérez, Jr., *Cuba under the Platt Amendment, 1902–1934* (Pittsburgh: University of Pittsburgh Press, 1986).

2. Joint Resolution of Congress for the Recognition of the Independence of Cuba, April 20, 1898, Congressional Record, 55th Cong., 2d Sess., 1898, 31:3988.

3. "La Convención Constituyente Cubana," *La Discusión* (Havana), July 21, 1900, 1.

4. Civil Order 301 in Leonard Wood, *Civil Report of Major General Leonard Wood, Military Governor of Cuba, (1900) for the Period from December 20th, 1899 to December 31st 1900,* 12 vols. (Washington: Government Printing Office, 1901). Also, in Spanish, Orden Número 301, July 25, 1900, in República de Cuba, Senado, *Memoria de los trabajos realizados durante las cuatro legislaturas y sesión extraordinaria del primer período congresional, 1902–1904* (Havana: Imprenta y Papelería de Rambla, Bouza y Ca., 1918), 151–52 (hereafter referred to as *Memoria*).

5. Civil Order 455 in Wood, *Civil Report of Major General Leonard Wood.* Also, in Spanish, "Alocución del Gobernador Militar de Cuba, leída en la apertura de la sesión inagural de la Convención Constituyente, el día 5 de noviembre de 1900," in República de Cuba, Senado, *Memoria,* 153–54.

6. Elihu Root to Leonard Wood, February 9, 1901, General Correspondence, 1901, Leonard Wood Papers, Manuscript Division, Library of Congress, Washington, DC.

7. Leonard Wood to Elihu Root, February 19, 1901, General Correspondence, 1901, Leonard Wood Papers.

8. Elihu Root to Leonard Wood, February 23, 1901, General Correspondence, 1901, Leonard Wood Papers.

9. Joint Resolution of Congress for the Recognition of the Independence of Cuba, April 20, 1898, Congressional Record, 55th Cong., 2d Sess., 1898, 31:3988.

10. Elihu Root to Leonard Wood, February 23, 1901, General Correspondence, 1901, Leonard Wood Papers.

11. The U.S. Supreme Court first recognized this point in *Gibbons v. Ogden,* 22 U.S. 1, 203 (1824). After reiterating that the states were completely sovereign and independent before the ratification of the U.S. Constitution in 1789, Chief Justice John Marshall wrote that the states continued to retain power over an "immense mass of legislation which embraces everything within the territory of a State not surrendered to the General Government; all which can be most advantageously exercised by the States themselves. Inspection laws, quarantine laws, health laws of every description . . . are component parts of this mass." In the *Slaughterhouse Cases,* 83 U.S. 36 (1872), the Supreme Court reaffirmed that even the sweeping changes brought about by the Civil War did not strip the states of their sovereign power to regulate health and sanitation.

12. Margaret Humphreys, *Yellow Fever and the South* (Baltimore: Johns Hopkins University Press, 1992), 13–14, 63–64.

13. Congressional Record, 56th Cong., 2nd Sess., 1901, 34: 3343.

14. Littlefield did not, however, go so far as to actually vote against the Platt Amendment; instead he abstained. See ibid., 3384.

15. *Neely v. Henkle,* 180 U.S. 109, 120 (1901).

16. Congressional Record, 56th Cong., 2nd Sess., 1901, 34: 3381.

17. Ibid., 3368.

18. Ibid., 3380.

19. Ibid., 3375.

20. Ibid., 3370.

21. Ibid., 3370.

22. Ibid., 3371.

23. Ibid.

24. Ibid., 3384.

25. Ibid., 3133.

26. Ibid., 3133–34.

27. Ibid., 3152.

28. Leonard Wood to Domingo Méndez Capote, March 2, 1901, in República de Cuba, Senado, *Memoria,* 423–24.

29. Elihu Root to Leonard Wood, February 25, 1901, General Correspondence, 1901, Leonard Wood Papers.

30. Acta de la Convención Constituyente, February 26, 1901, in República de Cuba, Senado, *Memoria,* 533.

31. Acta de la Convención Constituyente, March 7, 1901, *Memoria,* 538–41.

32. "Ponencia del Sr. Juan Gualberto Gómez, miembro de la comisión designada para proponer la respuesta a la comunicación del Gobernador Militar de Cuba," April 1, 1901, *Memoria,* 430.

33. "Proyecto de contestación a la comunicación del Gobernador Militar de Cuba, propuesto por el Delegado Sr. Eliseo Giberga," April 1, 1901, *Memoria,* 446–47.

34. Acta de la Convención Constituyente, April 13, 1901, *Memoria,* 560–63.

35. "Informe de la c[o]misión designada para avistarse con el gobierno de los Estados Unidos, dando cuenta del resultado de sus gestiones," May 7, 1901, *Memoria,* 478.

36. "Nuevo informe de la comisión designada para emitir dictamen sobre la Enmienda Platt, comunicada por el Gobernador Militar de Cuba," May 25, 1901, *Memoria,* 504.

37. "Apéndice a La Constitución de la República de Cuba," *La Discusión,* May 27, 1901.

38. Leonard Wood to Elihu Root, May 27, 1901, General Correspondence, 1901, Leonard Wood Papers.

39. Elihu Root to Leonard Wood, May 28, 1901, Outgoing Correspondence, Elihu Root Papers, Manuscript Division, Library of Congress, Washington, DC.

40. Acta de la Convención Constituyente, May 28, 1901, in República de Cuba, Senado, *Memoria,* 584–87.

41. "Cuban Problems Serious," *New York Times,* May 31, 1901.

42. "Cubans' Action Rejected," *New York Times,* June 1, 1901.

43. Elihu Root to Leonard Wood, May 31, 1901, Outgoing Correspondence, Elihu Root Papers.

44. "Topics of the Times," *New York Times,* June 10, 1901.

45. Leonard Wood to Domingo Méndez Capote, June 8, 1901, in República de Cuba, Senado, *Memoria,* 510–14.

46. Acta de la Convención Constituyente, June 12, 1901, in ibid., 591–93. Several of the delegates who were opposed to the Platt Amendment agreed not to attend the meeting. See "Cubans Preparing to Act," *New York Times,* June 12, 1901.

47. "The Cuban Way," *New York Times,* June 10, 1901, 6.

48. See, for example, "Our Relations with Cuba," *New York Times,* February 8, 1901, 6; and "No Action Yet at Havana," *New York Times,* February 23, 1901, 5.

49. "Disappointment in Cuba," *New York Times,* June 1, 1901, 1.

50. *New York Evening Post,* May 20, 1901.

51. "The Platt Amendment," *New York Times,* June 7, 1901.

52. Leonard Wood to the President and Congress of the Republic of Cuba, May 20, 1902, in United States Department of State, *Papers Relating to the Foreign Relations of the United States, with the Annual Message of the President Transmitted to Congress, December 1905* (Washington: Government Printing Office, 1906), 268.

53. Tomás Estrada Palma to Leonard Wood, May 20, 1902, in República de Cuba, Senado, *Memoria,* 789–90.

54. Tomás Estrada Palma, "Mensaje al Congreso de la República de Cuba," May 26, 1902, *Memoria,* 818.

55. Herbert G. Squiers to John Hay, June 2, 1902, Despatches from United States Ministers to Cuba, 1902–1906, General Records of the Department of State, Record Group 59, National Archives, Washington, DC (hereafter referred to as State/ RG 59).

56. Message of Tomás Estrada Palma, President of the Republic of Cuba, to the Congress of Cuba, May 26, 1902, Despatches from United States Ministers to Cuba, 1902–1906, State/ RG 59.

57. William C. Gorgas to William Forwood, Surgeon General U.S. Army, July 23, 1902, General Correspondence and Other Papers-I, 1902, William C. Gorgas Papers, Manuscript Division, Library of Congress, Washington, DC.

58. Tomás Estrada Palma, Message to the Congress of the Republic of Cuba, November 3, 1902, in United States Department of State, *Papers Relating to the Foreign Relations of the United States, with the Annual Message of the President Transmitted to Congress, December 2, 1902* (Washington: Government Printing Office, 1903), 347.

59. Report of Assistant Surgeon F. E. Trotter, in Marine-Hospital Service Treasury Department, *Annual Report of the Surgeon-General of the Public Health and Marine-Hospital Service of the United States for the Fiscal Year 1903* (Washington: Government Printing Office, 1904), 105.

60. Report of Assistant Surgeon R. H. von Ezdorf, August 11, 1903, in ibid., 112.

61. Report of Acting Assistant Surgeon E. F. McConnell, July 6, 1903, in ibid., 113.

62. Report of Acting Assistant Surgeon Richard Wilson, July 18, 1903, in ibid., 115.

63. Report of Acting Assistant Surgeon R. L. McMahon, June 30, 1903, in ibid., 119.

64. Report of Acting Assistant Surgeon E. F. Nuñez, July 8, 1904, in Marine-Hospital Service Treasury Department, *Annual Report of the Surgeon-General of the Public Health and Marine-Hospital Service of the United States for the Fiscal Year 1904* (Washington: Government Printing Office, 1904), 108.

65. Report of Acting Assistant Surgeon Richard Wilson, July 28, 1904, in ibid., 109–10.

66. Report of Acting Assistant Surgeon R. L. McMahon, July 1, 1904, in ibid., 114.

67. William W. Hadley to Herbert G. Squiers, October 15, 1904, Despatches from United States Ministers to Cuba, 1902–1906, State/ RG 59.

68. C. E. Little to Jacob Sleeper, October 26, 1904, Despatches from United States Ministers to Cuba, 1902–1906, State/ RG 59.

69. L. M. Shaw to John Hay, November 18, 1904, in Marine-Hospital Service Treasury Department, *Annual Report of the Surgeon-General of the Public Health and Marine-Hospital Service of the United States for the Fiscal Year 1905* (Washington: Government Printing Office, 1906), 50.

70. John Hay to Herbert G. Squiers, November 25, 1904, in United States Department of State, *Papers Relating to the Foreign Relations of the United States, with the Annual Message of the President Transmitted to Congress, December 6, 1904* (Washington: Government Printing Office, 1905), 251.

71. R. E. Holaday to Herbert G. Squiers, November 26, 1904, Despatches from United States Ministers to Cuba, 1902–1906, State/ RG 59.

72. Herbert G. Squiers to John Hay, November 28, 1904, Despatches from United States Ministers to Cuba, 1902–1906, State/ RG 59.

73. E. B. Webster to Herbert G. Squiers, November 30, 1904, Despatches from United States Ministers to Cuba, 1902–1906, State/ RG 59.

74. Raphaël Blanchard, *Les Moustiques: Histoire Naturelle et Médicale* (Paris: F.R. de Rudeval, 1905), 584.

75. "Nuestro estado sanitario," *La Lucha,* January 2, 1905, 1.

76. "Hay que defenderse," *La Lucha,* January 4, 1905, 2.

77. Herbert G. Squiers to John Hay, December 17, 1904, and Herbert G. Squiers to John Hay, January 14, 1905, Despatches from United States Ministers to Cuba, 1902–1906, State/ RG 59.

78. Treasury Department, *Annual Report of the Surgeon-General of the Public Health and Marine-Hospital Service of the United States for the Fiscal Year 1905,* 51–56.

79. Leonard Wood to the President and Congress of the Republic of Cuba, May 20, 1902, in United States Department of State, *Papers Relating to the Foreign Relations of the United States, with the Annual Message of the President Transmitted to Congress, December 1905,* 268.

80. John Hay to Herbert G. Squiers, March 10, 1905, in ibid., 267.

81. John Hay to Herbert G. Squiers, March 10, 1905, in ibid., 271.

82. See Herbert G. Squiers to Juan F. O'Farrill, March 31, 1905; Juan F. O'Farrill to Herbert G. Squiers, April 6, 1905; Acting Secretary of State Alvey A. Adee to Herbert G. Squiers, July 26, 1905; Herbert G. Squiers to Alvey A. Adee, August 17, 1905; and Secretary of State Elihu Root to Jacob Sleeper, December

21, 1905, Despatches from United States Ministers to Cuba, 1902–1906, State/ RG 59.

83. Tomás Estrada Palma, Message of the President of Cuba to the Cuban Congress, April 28, 1905, Despatches from United States Ministers to Cuba, 1902–1906, State/ RG 59.

84. Report of Passed Assistant Surgeon R. H. von Ezdorf, June 30, 1906, in Marine-Hospital Service Treasury Department, *Annual Report of the Surgeon-General of the Public Health and Marine-Hospital Service of the United States for the Fiscal Year 1906* (Washington: Government Printing Office, 1907), 77–79.

85. Report of Acting Assistant Surgeon E. F. Nuñez, June 30, 1906, in ibid., 80–82.

86. On the origin of the 1905 yellow fever epidemic in Havana, see General Report Presented by Drs. Hugo Roberts and Juan Guiteras, Delegates from Cuba, December 2, 1907, in International Sanitary Bureau of the American Republics, *Transaction of the Third International Sanitary Conference of the American Republics* (Washington: International Bureau of the American Republics, 1907), 162–66. For the Cuban government's position that the resolution of the epidemic in Havana demonstrated that the sanitary measures already in place were adequate, see Juan F. O'Farrill to Jacob Sleeper, January 10, 1906, Despatches from United States Ministers to Cuba, 1902–1906, State/ RG 59.

87. Elihu Root to Jacob Sleeper, January 20, 1906, in United States Department of State, *Papers Relating to the Foreign Relations of the United States, with the Annual Message of the President Transmitted to Congress, December 1906* (Washington: Government Printing Office, 1909), 506.

88. Juan F. O'Farrill to Jacob Sleeper, February 3, 1906, Despatches from United States Ministers to Cuba, 1902–1906, State/ RG 59.

89. Tomás Estrada Palma, Decree No. 224, June 6, 1906, and Edwin V. Morgan to Elihu Root, June 11, 1906, Despatches from United States Ministers to Cuba, 1902–1906, State/ RG 59.

90. For more on the political situation at this time see, David A. Lockmiller, *Magoon in Cuba: A History of the Second Intervention, 1906–1909* (Chapel Hill: University of North Carolina Press, 1938); Ibarra, *Cuba: 1898–1921, partidos políticos y clases sociales;* José M. Hernández, *Cuba and the United States: Intervention and Militarism, 1868–1933* (Austin: University of Texas Press, 1993); Pérez, *Cuba under the Platt Amendment, 1902–1934.*

91. William H. Taft to the People of Cuba, September 29, 1906, in Charles E. Magoon, *Republic of Cuba, Report of Provisional Administration from October 13th, 1906 to December 1st, 1907* (Havana: Rambla and Bouza, 1908), 5–6.

92. Report of Passed Assistant Surgeon J. W. Amesse, June 30, 1907, in Marine-Hospital Service Treasury Department, *Annual Report of the Surgeon-General of the Public Health and Marine-Hospital Service of the United States for the Fiscal Year 1907* (Washington: Government Printing Office, 1908), 75.

93. Magoon, *Republic of Cuba, Report of Provisional Administration from October 13th, 1906 to December 1st, 1907, 45.*

94. Report of Passed Assistant Surgeon J. W. Amesse, June 30, 1907, in Treasury Department, *Annual Report of the Surgeon-General of the Public Health and Marine-Hospital Service of the United States for the Fiscal Year 1907*, 74–75.

95. Report of Jefferson R. Kean, n.d., in Magoon, *Republic of Cuba, Report of Provisional Administration from October 13th, 1906 to December 1st, 1907*, 457.

96. Report of Passed Assistant Surgeon J. W. Amesse, June 30, 1908, in Marine-Hospital Service Treasury Department, *Annual Report of the Surgeon-General of the Public Health and Marine-Hospital Service of the United States for the Fiscal Year 1908* (Washington: Government Printing Office, 1909), 132.

97. Magoon, *Republic of Cuba, Report of Provisional Administration from October 13th, 1906 to December 1st, 1907*, 46.

98. A brief quarantine had been imposed against Havana in November 1905 and against Matanzas during the summer of 1906. For the Havana quarantine, see Report of Passed Assistant Surgeon R. H. von Ezdorf, June 30, 1906, in Treasury Department, *Annual Report of the Surgeon-General of the Public Health and Marine-Hospital Service of the United States for the Fiscal Year 1906*, 77. On the Matanzas quarantine, see Report of Acting Assistant Surgeon E. F. Nuñez, June 30, 1907, in Treasury Department, *Annual Report of the Surgeon-General of the Public Health and Marine-Hospital Service of the United States for the Fiscal Year 1907*, 75.

99. Report of Passed Assistant Surgeon J. W. Amesse, June 30, 1907, in Treasury Department, *Annual Report of the Surgeon-General of the Public Health and Marine-Hospital Service of the United States for the Fiscal Year 1907*, 74.

100. George B. Cortelyou to William H. Taft, December 6, 1907, File 209, "Confidential" Correspondence, 1906–1909, Records of the Provisional Government of Cuba, Record Group 199, National Archives, College Park, Maryland (hereafter referred to as PGC/RG 199).

101. Charles E. Magoon to William H. Taft, December 10, 1907, File 209, "Confidential" Correspondence, 1906–1909, PGC/RG 199.

102. Report of Jefferson R. Kean, n.d., in Magoon, *Republic of Cuba, Report of Provisional Administration from October 13th, 1906 to December 1st, 1907*, 456. The original members of the Board were Carlos J. Finlay, Juan Guiteras, Enrique Nuñez, J. A. López del Valle, Emilio del Junco, Rogelio Espinosa, and Enrique B. Barnet. Report of Enrique B. Barnet, October 31, 1908, in Charles E. Magoon, *Republic of Cuba, Report of Provisional Administration from December 1st, 1907 to December 1st, 1908* (Havana: Rambla and Bouza, 1909), 447.

103. Magoon, *Republic of Cuba, Report of Provisional Administration from October 13th, 1906 to December 1st, 1907*, 459.

104. Report of Carlos J. Finlay, November 10, 1908, in Magoon, *Republic of Cuba, Report of Provisional Administration from December 1st, 1907 to December 1st, 1908*, 442–43.

105. Treasury Department, *Annual Report of the Surgeon-General of the*

Public Health and Marine-Hospital Service of the United States for the Fiscal Year 1908, 97.

106. Jefferson R. Kean to John N. Thomas, Acting Assistant Surgeon, U.S. Marine Hospital Service, March 26, 1908, File 209, "Confidential" Correspondence, 1906–1909, PGC/RG 199.

107. Charles E. Magoon to Clarence R. Edwards, Chief of Bureau of Insular Affairs, March 29, 1908, File 209, "Confidential" Correspondence, 1906–1909, PGC/RG 199.

108. Treasury Department, *Annual Report of the Surgeon-General of the Public Health and Marine-Hospital Service of the United States for the Fiscal Year 1908*, 97.

109. Report of Jefferson R. Kean, Adviser to Sanitary Department, November 10, 1908, in Magoon, *Republic of Cuba, Report of Provisional Administration from December 1st, 1907 to December 1st, 1908*, 437–38.

110. Treasury Department, *Annual Report of the Surgeon-General of the Public Health and Marine-Hospital Service of the United States for the Fiscal Year 1908*, 98.

111. Report of Jefferson R. Kean, Adviser to Sanitary Department, November 10, 1908, in Magoon, *Republic of Cuba, Report of Provisional Administration from December 1st, 1907 to December 1st, 1908*, 437–38; Treasury Department, *Annual Report of the Surgeon-General of the Public Health and Marine-Hospital Service of the United States for the Fiscal Year 1908*, 98.

112. Report of Enrique B. Barnet, October 31, 1908, in Magoon, *Republic of Cuba, Report of Provisional Administration from December 1st, 1907 to December 1st, 1908*, 447–64.

113. Report of Carlos J. Finlay, November 10, 1908, in ibid., 443.

114. Charles E. Magoon to the Congress of the Republic of Cuba, January 28, 1909, in United States Congress. Senate, *Supplemental Report of Provisional Governor of Cuba*, 61st Congress, 1st Session, No. 80, Ser. 5572 (Washington: Government Printing Office, 1909), 27.

115. Magoon, *Republic of Cuba, Report of Provisional Administration from December 1st, 1907 to December 1st, 1908*, 143.

116. Ibid.

117. Magoon, *Republic of Cuba, Report of Provisional Administration from October 13th, 1906 to December 1st, 1907*, 459.

118. Magoon, *Republic of Cuba, Report of Provisional Administration from December 1st, 1907 to December 1st, 1908*, 143–44. The yellow fever point was considered to be when there was more than one mosquito for each 1000 houses inspected. Jefferson R. Kean to Charles E. Magoon, June 3, 1908, File 171, "Confidential" Correspondence, 1906–1909, PGC/RG 199.

119. Report of D. Lombillo Clark, October 30, 1908, in Magoon, *Republic of Cuba, Report of Provisional Administration from December 1st, 1907 to December 1st, 1908*, 352–88.

120. Charles E. Magoon to the President and Congress of the Republic of Cuba, January 28, 1909, in United States Congress. Senate, *Supplemental Report of Provisional Governor of Cuba*, 9.

121. Translation of article in *El Cubano Libre,* May 14, 1907, File 127, "Confidential" Correspondence, 1906–1909, PGC/RG 199.

122. Pazos, "Contribución al estudio de los mosquitos en Cuba," *Sanidad y beneficiencia* 2, no. 1 (1909): 28.

123. The quote comes from Jefferson R. Kean to Charles E. Magoon, June 3, 1908, File 171, "Confidential" Correspondence, 1906–1909, PGC/RG 199.

CHAPTER 6

1. Antonio Gramsci, *Selections from the Prison Notebooks,* trans. Quintin Hoare and Geoffrey Nowell-Smith (New York: International Publishers, 1971).

2. Frantz Fanon, *A Study in Dying Colonialism,* trans. Haakon Chevalier (New York: Grove Press, 1965), 122.

3. Octave Mannoni, *Prospero and Caliban: The Psychology of Colonization,* trans. Pamela Powesland (New York: Frederick A. Praeger, 1956), 47.

4. Albert Memmi, *Portrait du colonisé* (Paris: Gallimard, 1985), 101.

5. Writing in 1955, Aimé Césaire warned the colonized nations of Africa, Asia, and the West Indies that their situations could not be improved by substituting the United States for their old European rulers: "I know that some of you, disgusted with Europe . . . are turning . . . towards America and getting used to looking upon that country as a possible liberator. . . . The bulldozers! The massive investment of capital! The roads! The ports! . . . But American racism! . . . American domination—the only domination from which one never recovers. I mean from which one never recovers unscarred." Aimé Césaire, *Discourse on Colonialism,* trans. Joan Pinkham (New York: Monthly Review Press, 1972), 60.

6. Manuel Delfín, *La Higiene* 1, no. 24 (August 30, 1900): 1.

7. For information on the U.S. demands of Cuban gratitude, see Louis A. Pérez, Jr., "Incurring a Debt of Gratitude: 1898 and the Moral Sources of United States Hegemony in Cuba," *American Historical Review* 104, no. 2 (1999). On U.S. Army treatment of the Cuban Liberation Army, see Louis A. Pérez, Jr., *Cuba between Empires, 1878–1902* (Pittsburgh: University of Pittsburgh Press, 1983), 196–210.

8. José Manuel Espin, "Paludismo, fiebre amarilla y filariasis: Doctrina moderna de la transmisión de estas enfermedades por los mosquitos," *Sanidad y beneficiencia* 4, no. 1 (1910): 110.

9. "May Be Duel in Cabinet: One Member of Cuban Ministry Challenges Another to Fight," *New York Times,* October 23, 1909, 10; "Notes of Foreign Affairs," *New York Times,* January 22, 1910, C4.

10. "The Cuban Menace," *Medical Record* 75 (June 5, 1909): 975.

11. Quoted in *Army and Navy Journal,* October 1, 1910.

12. "Sanitary Neglect in Cuba a Menace: Gomez Government Has Allowed Campaign against Yellow Fever to Drop," *New York Times,* May 28, 1909, 4.

13. *Army and Navy Journal,* October 1, 1910.

14. Ibid.

15. Matías Duque, "To the Medical Record," *Sanidad y beneficiencia* 1, no. 3 (1909): 348, 346.

16. Ibid., 345.

17. Ibid., 346.

18. Ibid., 347.

19. Ibid., 347–48. Upon receiving Duque's letter, the editors of the *Medical Record* expressed their pleasure in learning that the sanitary conditions in Cuba were in such a good state, but they continued to argue that the situation was bound to get worse unless the Cuban politicians were supervised: "The danger is, as we have maintained, that the needs of the politicians may hamper the work of the health department and impair its efficiency. What has happened before may happen again if those in control of the government forget their responsibility in sanitary matters." The problem of keeping politicians focused on public health needs was not unique to Cuba, the *Record* acknowledged, "but it happens that just now, and for the hot months to come, it is this country that will suffer if the Cuban authorities are not alive to their duty to themselves and to us." Any hint of deterioration in the sanitation of Havana would be seen as a threat to the United States. "Sanitary Conditions in Cuba," *Medical Record* 75 (June 19, 1909): 1062.

20. Juan Guiteras to the editor of the *Army and Navy Journal*, December 25, 1910, in "An Article from the 'Army and Navy Journal' and Reply of the Director of Public Health," *Sanidad y beneficiencia* 5, no. 1 (1911): 80–81.

21. Juan Guiteras, "The Supression of Yellow Fever in Cuba," *Medical Record* 75 (June 26, 1909): 1109.

22. Matías Duque, "Cuba," *Sanidad y beneficiencia* 2, no. 2 (1909): 120.

23. Ibid., 123.

24. Ibid., 125.

25. José A. López del Valle, "La lucha contra el mosquito: Empleo de medios auxiliares, las biajacas, los guajacones," *Sanidad y beneficiencia* 3, no. 3 (1910): 224–26.

26. Gabriel Custodio, "Contribution to the Study of the Technique of Fumigations," *Sanidad y beneficiencia* 3, nos. 1 and 2 (1910): 33.

27. Juan Guiteras, "A False Alarm of Yellow Fever and How It Was Met by the Health Department," *Sanidad y beneficiencia* 6, nos. 5 and 6 (1911): 664.

28. Ibid., 664–66.

29. Juan Guiteras, "La sanidad cubana y la opinión extranjera," *Sanidad y beneficiencia* 2, no. 1 (1909): 1.

30. Ibid.

31. Juan Guiteras to the editor of the *Army and Navy Journal*, December 25, 1910, in "An Article from the 'Army and Navy Journal' and Reply of the Director of Public Health," *Sanidad y beneficiencia* 5, no. 1 (1911): 80–81.

32. Arístides Agramonte, "Yellow Fever Profilaxis in Cuba," *Medical Record* 76 (September 4, 1909): 394.

33. Ibid., 398–99.

34. Ibid., 399.

35. *La Discusión,* February 22, 1910. To the island's sanitarians, the ob-

servation hurt like the truth. Guiteras tried to soothe the sting by arguing that the fight against yellow fever was waged not just for the United States, but also for "the regard for humanity, the regard for the good name of our people, and the upbuilding of a strong and capable race" through increases in immigration. Juan Guiteras, "Tuberculosis in Cuba," *Sanidad y beneficiencia* 3, nos. 1 and 2 (1910): 8–9. For a discussion of the relative severity of yellow fever and tuberculosis in Cuba, see chapter 4.

36. Espin, "Paludismo, fiebre amarilla y filariasis: Doctrina moderna de la transmisión de estas enfermedades por los mosquitos," 105.

37. Walter Reed to Jefferson Randolph Kean, September 25, 1900, File 02125001, Walter Reed Series, Philip S. Hench Walter Reed Yellow Fever Collection, University of Virginia, Charlottesville, VA. Lazear's letters to his wife, however, reveal that Reed and James Carroll took little or no interest in Lazear's work and that he was keeping his findings secret from them. Jesse W. Lazear to Mabel H. Lazear, July 15, 1900, File 003340001; Jesse W. Lazear to Mabel H. Lazear, August 23, 1900, File 003410001; Jesse W. Lazear to Mabel H. Lazear, September 8, 1900, File 003440001; all in Jesse W. Lazear Series, Philip S. Hench Walter Reed Yellow Fever Collection, University of Virginia, Charlottesville, VA. See chapter 3 for a detailed discussion of the work of the Yellow Fever Commission in Cuba during 1900.

38. William C. Gorgas to Walter Reed, February 6, 1902, File 02604001, Walter Reed Series, Philip S. Hench Walter Reed Yellow Fever Collection. Gorgas indignantly quoted Reed's words in this letter. He assured Reed that his "name will be remembered in medicine with Jenner & Wills long after the old doctor has been forgotten so do not begrudge the old man his little need of praise."

39. Juan Guiteras, "Conferencia del Dr. Osler sobre "La Nación y los Trópicos" y el Dr. Finlay," *Sanidad y beneficiencia* 3, no. 4 (1910): 317.

40. Espin, "Paludismo, fiebre amarilla y filariasis: Doctrina moderna de la transmisión de estas enfermedades por los mosquitos," 111.

41. Ibid., 113–14.

42. Paulsor, "La conquista científica de la fiebre amarilla," *Sanidad y beneficiencia* 5, no. 1 (1911): 108.

43. "Comentario: La conquista científica de la fiebre amarilla," *Sanidad y beneficiencia* 5, no. 2 (1911): 256.

44. Ibid.

45. José A. López del Valle, "Al Congreso de la Prensa Médica Latina," *Sanidad y beneficiencia* 32, nos. 1, 2, and 3 (1927): 202.

46. Jorge Le-Roy, "Reivindicación de la Gloria de Finlay," *Sanidad y beneficiencia* 32, nos. 1, 2, and 3 (1927): 204.

47. Ibid., 215.

48. Juan Guiteras, "El Dr. Carlos J. Finlay: Apuntes biográficos," *Anales de la Academia de Ciencias Médicas, Físicas y Naturales de La Habana* 48 (1911): 271.

49. Juan Santos Fernández, "Contestación al discurso de recepción del Dr. Juan Guiteras en la Academia de Ciencias," *Anales de la Academia de Ciencias Médicas, Físicas y Naturales de La Habana* 48 (October 1911): 284–85.

50. Ibid., 281.

51. Ibid., 282.

52. José A. López del Valle, "Discurso por el Dr. J. A. López del Valle, Secretario de la Junta Nacional de Sanidad y Beneficiencia y Profesor de Higiene de la Universidad Nacional, en el acto de desvelar las tarjas con los nombres de Finlay y de Guiteras," *Sanidad y beneficiencia* 32, nos. 1, 2, and 3 (1927): 164.

53. Ibid.

54. Ibid., 166.

55. Ibid. The Finlay Institute developed much as López del Valle envisioned. By the 1980s, it was the core of Cuban efforts to develop biotechnological advances suiting the needs of developing countries; in this role, it served explicitly as a symbol of both Cuban scientific achievement and resistance to U.S. domination. See Simon Reid-Henry, *The Cuban Cure: Reason and Resistance in Global Science* (Chicago: University of Chicago Press, 2009).

56. López del Valle, "Discurso por el Dr. J. A. López del Valle, Secretario de la Junta Nacional de Sanidad y Beneficiencia y Profesor de Higiene de la Universidad Nacional, en el acto de desvelar las tarjas con los nombres de Finlay y de Guiteras," 167.

CHAPTER 7

1. William C. Gorgas, "Sanitary Conditions as Encountered in Cuba and Panama, and What Is Being Done to Render the Canal Zone Healthy," read before the Fourth Pan American Medical Congress, Panama, January 3–4, 1905, and printed in the *Medical Record,* February 4, 1905, Addresses, Articles, and Reports, 1901–12 and Undated, William C. Gorgas Papers, Manuscript Division, Library of Congress, Washington, DC.

2. William C. Gorgas to the Secretary of War, "Sanitation of Guayaquil," January 9, 1913, Yellow Fever-Miscellaneous Papers, William C. Gorgas Papers.

3. For further discussion on the role of entomologists and the understanding of tropical environments in the Panama Canal, see Paul S. Sutter, "Nature's Agents or Agents of Empire? Entomological Workers and Environmental Change during the Construction of the Panama Canal," *Isis* 98, no. 4 (2007): 724–54.

4. International Health Commission Resolution, May, 1915, in Andrew J. Warren, "Landmarks in the Conquest of Yellow Fever," in *Yellow Fever,* ed. George K. Strode, et al. (New York: McGraw-Hill Book Co., 1951), 14. See also Juan Guiteras, "The Panama Canal and the Propagation of Epidemic Diseases," *Sanidad y beneficiencia* 6, no. 2 (1911): 220–21.

5. Warren, "Landmarks in the Conquest of Yellow Fever," 12–13.

6. Henry R. Carter to William C. Gorgas, "Report on Yellow Fever in Guayaquil," July 20, 1916, File 00807022, Henry R. Carter Series, Philip S. Hench Walter Reed Yellow Fever Collection, the Claude Moore Health Sciences Library, University of Virginia, Charlottesville, VA.

7. William C. Gorgas to the Secretary of War, "Sanitation of Guayaquil,"

January 9, 1913, Yellow Fever-Miscellaneous Papers, William C. Gorgas Papers.

8. "A Sanitary Campaign," *New York Times,* October 13, 1916, 10.

9. Henry R. Carter, "Lecture on the Prophylaxis of Yellow Fever," n.d. (1922–23), File 01006001, Henry R. Carter Series, Philip S. Hench Walter Reed Yellow Fever Collection.

10. For more information on the Rockefeller Foundation in Latin America, see Marcos Cueto, ed., *Missionaries of Science: The Rockefeller Foundation and Latin America* (Bloomington: Indiana University Press, 1994). For the present extent of endemic yellow fever in South America, see Map 4–16 in Centers for Disease Control and Prevention, *Health Information for International Travel 2008* (Atlanta: US Department of Health and Human Services, Public Health Service, 2007).

Bibliography

ARCHIVES CONSULTED

Archivo Nacional de Cuba, Havana, Cuba
    Junta Superior de Sanidad (1839–1907)
    Secretaría de Estado y Gobernación (1899–1902)
Biblioteca Nacional José Martí, Havana, Cuba
    Colección de Publicaciones Seriadas
Museo de Historia de las Ciencias en Cuba "Carlos J. Finlay,"
    Havana, Cuba
National Archives of the United States, College Park,
    Maryland
    Records of the American Red Cross. Record Group 200
    Records of the Bureau of Insular Affairs. Record Group
        350
    Records of the Military Government of Cuba. Record
        Group 140 (Note: the file numbers for Letters Re-
        ceived, 1899–1902, are created by author to facilitate
        finding alphabetical files in boxes.)
    Records of the Provisional Government of Cuba. Record
        Group 199
    Records of the Public Health Service. Record Group 90
National Archives of the United States, Washington, D.C.
    Records of the Department of State. Record Group 59
Library of Congress, Washington, D.C.
    George B. Cortelyou Papers
    William C. Gorgas Papers
    William McKinley Papers
    Elihu Root Papers
    Leonard Wood Papers

Philip S. Hench Walter Reed Yellow Fever Collection, Claude Moore Health
  Sciences Library, University of Virginia, Charlottesville, Virginia
    Diplomas and Certificates
    Jefferson Randolph Kean Series
    Jesse W. Lazear Series
    Walter Reed Series
    Edward Hook Additions
    James Carroll Papers
Orville H. Platt Papers, Connecticut State Library, Hartford, Connecticut
Carlos Finlay Collection, Scott Memorial Library, Thomas Jefferson University,
  Philadelphia, Pennsylvania

NEWSPAPERS

Atlanta Constitution
Chicago Daily Tribune
La Discusión (Havana)
Brooklyn Eagle
Galveston Daily News
Houston Daily Post
Jackson Daily Bulletin
Jackson Daily Clarion-Ledger
La Lucha (Havana)
Los Angeles Times
El Imparcial (Madrid)
New Orleans Daily Picayune
New York Daily Tribune
New York Herald
New York Journal
New York News
New York Sun
New York Times

PUBLISHED SOURCES

Agramonte, Arístides. "Yellow Fever Profilaxis in Cuba." *Medical Record* 76
  (September 4, 1909): 394–99.
Anderson, Warwick. *Colonial Pathologies: American Tropical Medicine, Race,
  and Hygiene in the Philippines.* Durham: Duke University Press, 2006.
———. "Disease, Race, and Empire." *Bulletin of the History of Medicine* 70,
  no. 1 (1996): 62–67.
———. "Excremental Colonialism: Public Health and the Poetics of Pollution." *Critical Inquiry* 21, no. 3 (1995): 640–69.
———. "Immunities of Empire: Race, Disease, and the New Tropical Medicine, 1900–1920." *Bulletin of the History of Medicine* 70, no. 1 (1996):
  94–118.

―――. "Leprosy and Citizenship." *Positions: East Asia Cultures Critique* 6, no. 3 (1998): 707–30.

Armus, Diego, ed. *Disease in the History of Latin America: From Malaria to AIDS.* Durham: Duke University Press, 2003.

―――. "Salud y anarquía: La tuberculosis en el discurso libertario argentino, 1890–1940."

Army and Navy Journal (October 1, 1910).

Arnold, David. "Cholera and Colonialism in British India." *Past and Present* 113 (1986): 118–51.

―――. *Colonizing the Body: State Medicine and Epidemic Disease in Nineteenth-Century India.* Berkeley: University of California Press, 1993.

―――. *Science, Technology, and Medicine in Colonial India.* Cambridge: Cambridge University Press, 2000.

Ashby, Roland Rieder, and Charlotte M. Ashby. "Preliminary Inventory of the Records of the Provisional Government of Cuba (Record Group 199)." Washington: National Archives, 1962.

Ashford, Bailey K. *A Soldier in Science.* New York: William Morrow and Co., 1934.

Balke, Nathan S., and Robert J. Gordon. "The Estimation of Prewar Gross National Product: Methodology and New Evidence." *Journal of Political Economy* 97, no. 1 (1989): 38–92.

Bangs, John Kendrick. *Uncle Sam Trustee.* New York: Riggs Publishing Co., 1901.

Bean, William B. "Walter Reed and Yellow Fever." *Journal of the American Medical Association* 250, no. 5 (1983): 659–62.

Benchimol, Jaime Larry. *Dos micróbios aos mosquitos: Febre amarela e a revolução pausteriana no Brasil.* Rio de Janeiro: Universidade Federal do Rio de Janeiro, 1999.

Benjamin, Jules R. *The United States and Cuba: Hegemony and Dependent Development, 1880–1934.* Pittsburgh: University of Pittsburgh Press, 1977.

―――. *The United States and the Origins of the Cuban Revolution: An Empire of Liberty in an Age of National Liberation.* Princeton: Princeton University Press, 1990.

Birn, Anne-Emanuelle. "Revolution, the Scatological Way: The Rockefeller Foundation's Hookworm Campaign in 1920s Mexico." In *Disease in the History of Latin America: From Malaria to AIDS,* edited by Diego Armus. Durham: Duke University Press, 2003.

Blanchard, Raphaël. *Les Moustiques: Histoire naturelle et médicale.* Paris: F. R. de Rudeval, 1905.

Bloom, Kahled J. *The Mississippi Valley's Great Yellow Fever Epidemic of 1878.* Baton Rouge: Louisiana State University Press, 1993.

Blum, Edward. "The Crucible of Disease: Trauma, Memory, and National Reconciliation during the Yellow Fever Epidemic of 1878." *Journal of Southern History* 69, no. 4 (2003): 791–820.

Bonsal, Stephen. "The real condition of Cuba to-day." *Review of Reviews* 15, no. 5 (1897): 562–76.

Bradford, James C. "Introduction." In *Crucible of Empire: The Spanish-*

American War and Its Aftermath, edited by James C. Bradford. Annapolis: Naval Institute Press, 1993.

Bretelle-Establet, Florence. "Resistance and Receptivity: French Colonial Medicine in Southwest China, 1898–1930." *Modern China* 25, no. 2 (1999): 171–203.

Briggs, Asa. "Cholera and Society in the Nineteenth Century." *Past and Present* 19 (1961): 76–96.

Brock, Thomas D. *Robert Koch, A Life in Medicine and Bacteriology.* Madison: Science Tech Publishers, 1988.

Brooke, John R. *Civil Report of Major-General John R. Brooke, U.S. Army, Military Governor of Cuba: 1899.* Washington: Government Printing Office, 1900.

Brown, E. Richard. "Public Health in Imperialism: Early Rockefeller Programs at Home and Abroad." *American Journal of Public Health* 66, no. 9 (1976): 896–903.

Brunner, W. F. "Morbidity and Mortality in the Spanish Army During the Calendar Year 1897." *Public Health Reports* 13, no. 17 (April 29, 1898).

———. "Sanitary Report from Habana." *Public Health Reports* 12, no. 34 (August 20, 1897).

———. "Sanitary Report from Habana." *Public Health Reports* 12, no. 39 (September 24, 1897).

Burke, Timothy. *Lifebuoy Men, Lux Women: Commodification, Consumption, and Cleanliness in Modern Zimbabwe.* Durham: Duke University Press, 1996.

Byerly, Carol R. *Fever of War: The Influenza Epidemic in the U.S. Army during World War I.* New York: New York University Press, 2005.

Carrigan, Jo Ann. "Privilege, Prejudice, and the Strangers' Disease in Nineteenth-Century New Orleans." *Journal of Southern History* 36, no. 4 (1970): 568–78.

———. *The Saffron Scourge: A History of Yellow Fever in Louisiana, 1796–1905.* Lafayette: Center for Louisiana Studies, University of Southwestern Louisiana, 1994.

Carter, Henry R. "A Note on the Interval between Infecting and Secondary Cases of Yellow Fever from the Records of the Yellow Fever at Orwood and Taylor, Miss., in 1898." *New Orleans Medical and Surgical Journal* 52, no. 11 (1900): 618–36.

———. *Yellow Fever: An Epidemiological and Historical Study of Its Place of Origin.* Baltimore: Williams and Wilkins Co., 1931.

Centers for Disease Control and Prevention. *Health Information for International Travel 2008.* Atlanta: US Department of Health and Human Services, Public Health Service, 2007.

Césaire, Aimé. *Discourse on Colonialism.* Translated by Joan Pinkham. New York: Monthly Review Press, 1972.

Chaillé, Stanford E. "Report to the United States National Board of Health on Yellow Fever in Havana and Cuba." In *Annual Report of the National Board of Health, 1880,* edited by U.S. National Board of Health. Washington: Government Printing Office, 1881.

Chevalier, Louis. *Le choléra, la première épidémie du XIXe siècle.* La Roche-sur-Yon: Imprimerie Centrale de l'Ouest, 1958.

Cirillo, Vincent J. *Bullets and Bacilli: The Spanish-American War and Military Medicine.* New Bruswick: Rutgers University Press, 2004.

———. "'The Patriotic Odor': Sanitation and Typhoid Fever in the National Encampments during the Spanish-American War." *Army History: The Professional Bulletin of Army History* 20–00–2, no. 49 (2000): 17–23.

Cliff, Andrew, Peter Haggett, and Matthew Smallman-Raynor. *Deciphering Global Epidemics: Analytical Approaches to the Disease Records of World Cities, 1888–1912.* Cambridge: Cambridge University Press, 1998.

Coelho, Philip R. P., and Robert A. McGuire. "African and European Bound Labor in the British New World: The Biological Consequences of Economic Choices." *Journal of Economic History* 57, no. 1 (1997): 83–115.

Cohen, William B. "Malaria and French Imperialism." *Journal of African History* 24, no. 1 (1983): 23–36.

Coleman, William. *Yellow Fever in the North: The Methods of Early Epidemiology.* Madison: University of Wisconsin Press, 1987.

"Comentario: La conquista científica de la fiebre amarilla." *Sanidad y beneficiencia* 5, no. 2 (1911): 256.

Comité Guatemalteco Pro-Centenario Finlay y Día de la Medicina Americana. *La fiebre amarilla en Guatemala: Homenaje al Doctor Carlos J. Finlay en el primer centenario de su nacimiento: 3 de diciembre de 1933.* Guatemala: Universidad Nacional de Guatemala, 1933.

Cook, Noble David. *Born to Die: Disease and New World Conquest, 1492–1650.* Cambridge: Cambridge University Press, 1998.

Cooper, Donald B. "The New "Black Death": Cholera in Brazil, 1855–1856." *Social Science History* 10, no. 4 (1986): 467–88.

Cooper, Frederick, and Ann Laura Stoler, eds. *Tensions of Empire: Colonial Culture in a Bourgeois World.* Berkeley: University of California Press, 1997.

Cosmas, Graham A. "Securing the Fruits of Victory: The U.S. Army Occupies Cuba, 1898–1899." *Military Affairs* 38, no. 3 (1974): 85–91.

Craddock, Wallis Landes. "The Achievements of William Crawford Gorgas." *Military Medicine* 162, no. 5 (1997): 325–27.

Crosby, Alfred W. *Ecological Imperialism: The Biological Expansion of Europe, 900–1900.* Cambridge: Cambridge University Press, 1986.

———. *Epidemic and Peace, 1918.* Westport: Greenwood Press, 1976.

———. *The Columbian Exchange: Biological and Cultural Consequences of 1492.* Westport: Greenwood Publishing Co., 1972.

Crosby, Molly Caldwell. *The American Plague: The Untold Story of Yellow Fever, the Epidemic That Shaped Our History.* New York: Berkley Books, 2006.

Cueto, Marcos. *Cold War, Deadly Fevers: Malaria Eradication in Mexico, 1955–1975.* Baltimore: Johns Hopkins University Press, 2007.

———, ed. *Missionaries of Science: The Rockefeller Foundation and Latin America.* Bloomington: Indiana University Press, 1994.

———, ed. *Salud, cultura y sociedad en América Latina.* Lima: Instituto de Estudios Peruanos, 1996.

————. "Sanitation from Above: Yellow Fever and Foreign Intervention in Peru, 1919–1922." *Hispanic American Historical Review* 72, no. 1 (1992): 1–22.

————. *The Return of Epidemics: Health and Society in Peru during the Twentieth Century.* Aldershot, UK: Ashgate Publishing, 2001.

————. *The Value of Health: A History of the Pan American Health Organization.* Washington: Pan American Health Organization, 2007.

Cummins, Lejeune. "The Formulation of the Platt Amendment." *The Americas* 23, no. 4 (1967): 370–88.

Curtin, Philip D. *Death by Migration: Europe's Encounter with the Tropical World in the Nineteenth Century.* Cambridge: Cambridge University Press, 1989.

————. *Disease and Empire: The Health of European Troops in the Conquest of Africa.* Cambridge: Cambridge University Press, 1998.

————. *The Image of Africa: British Ideas and Actions, 1780–1850.* Madison: University of Wisconsin Press, 1964.

Curtis, William Elroy. "Cuba and Her People." *Chatauquant* 27, no. May (1898): 185–90.

Custodio, Gabriel. "Contribution to the Study of the Technique of Fumigations." *Sanidad y beneficiencia* 3, no. 1 and 2 (1910): 31–33.

Davey, Richard. *Cuba, Past and Present.* New York: Charles Scribner's Sons, 1898.

Davis, Richard Harding. *Cuba in War Time.* New York: R. H. Russell, 1897.

De Barros, Juanita. *Order and Place in a Colonial City: Patterns of Struggle and Resistance in Georgetown, British Guiana, 1889–1924.* Montreal and Kingston: McGill-Queen's University Press, 2002.

de Diego, Emilio. *1895: La Guerra en Cuba y la España de la Restauración,* Cursos de Verano de el Escorial. Moreto: Editorial Complutense, S. A., 1996.

de Kruif, Paul. *Microbe Hunters.* New York: Harcourt, Brace, and Co., 1926.

de Larra y Cerezo, Ángel. *Datos para la historia de la campaña sanitaria en la Guerra de Cuba: Apuntes estadísticos relativos del año 1896.* Madrid: Imprenta de Ricardo Rojas, 1901.

Del Regato, Juan Ángel. "Carlos Finlay and the Carrier of Death: The Cycle of Successful Scientific Discovery." *Jefferson Medical College Alumni Bulletin* (1971): 1–16.

Delaporte, François. *The History of Yellow Fever: An Essay on the Birth of Tropical Medicine.* Translated by Arthur Goldhammer. Cambridge: MIT Press, 1991.

Delfín, Manuel. *La higiene* 1, no. 24 (August 30, 1900): 1–2.

————. *Nociones de higiene.* Havana: Imprenta "La Propagandista," 1901.

Diamond, Jared M. *Guns, Germs, and Steel: The Fates of Human Societies.* New York: W. W. Norton and Co., 1997.

Dorfman, Ariel. *The Empire's Old Clothes: What the Lone Ranger, Babar, and Other Innocent Heroes Do to Our Minds.* New York: Pantheon Books, 1983.

Duffy, John. *Sword of Pestilence: The New Orleans Yellow Fever Epidemic of 1853.* Baton Rouge: Louisiana State University Press, 1966.

Duffy, Michael. *Soldiers, Sugar, and Seapower: The British Expeditions to the West Indies and the War against Revolutionary France.* Oxford: Oxford University Press, 1987.

Dumett, Raymond E. "The Campaign against Malaria and the Expansion of Scientific Medical and Sanitary Services in British West Africa, 1898–1910." *African Historical Studies* 1, no. 2 (1968): 153–97.

Duque, Matías. "Cuba." *Sanidad y beneficiencia* 2, no. 2 (1909): 119–25.

———. "To the Medical Record." *Sanidad y beneficiencia* 1, no. 3 (1909): 345–48.

Echenberg, Myron. *Black Death, White Medicine: Bubonic Plague and the Politics of Public Health in Colonial Senegal, 1914–1945.* Portsmouth, NH: Heinemann, 2002.

Eigenmann. "Yellow Fever and Fishes in Colombia." *Proceedings of the American Philosophical Society* 63, no. 3 (1924): 236–38.

Ellis, John H. *Yellow Fever and Public Health in the New South.* Lexington: University Press of Kentucky, 1992.

Espin, José Manuel. "Paludismo, fiebre amarilla y filariasis: Doctrina moderna de la transmisión de estas enfermedades por los mosquitos." *Sanidad y beneficiencia* 4, no. 1 (1910): 105137.

Ettling, John. *The Germ of Laziness: Rockefeller Philanthropy and Public Health in the New South.* Cambridge: Harvard University Press, 1981.

Evans, Richard J. "Epidemics and Revolutions: Cholera in Nineteenth-Century Europe." *Past and Present* 120 (1988): 123–46.

Fanon, Frantz. *A Study in Dying Colonialism.* Translated by Haakon Chevalier. New York: Grove Press, 1965.

Fernández, Susan J. *Encumbered Cuba: Capital Markets and Revolt, 1878–1895.* Gainesville: University Press of Florida, 2002.

Fernós, Rodrigo. *Medicine and International Relations in the Caribbean: Some Historical Variants.* New York: iUniverse, 2006.

Finlay, Carlos J. "El mosquito hipotéticamente considerado como agente de transmisión de la fiebre amarilla." *Anales de la Academia de Ciencias Médicas, Físicas y Naturales de La Habana* 18 (1881): 147–69.

———. *Estudios sobre la fiebre amarilla.* Havana: Publicaciones del Ministerio de Educación, 1945.

———. *Obras Completas.* Havana: Academia de Ciencias de Cuba, 1965.

Foner, Philip S. *The Spanish-Cuban-American War and the Birth of American Imperialism, 1895–1902.* 2 vols. New York: Monthly Review Press, 1972.

Fraga, Clementino. *A febre amarela no Brasil; Nota e documentos de uma grande campanha sanitaria.* Rio de Janeiro: Off. Graph. da Insp. de Demografia Sanitária, 1930.

Franklin, Jon, and John Sutherland. *Guinea Pig Doctors: The Drama of Medical Research through Self-Experimentation.* New York: William Morrow and Co., 1984.

Freidel, Frank. *The Splendid Little War.* Boston: Little Brown, 1958.

Freund, Peter E. S. *The Civilized Body: Social Domination, Control, and Health.* Philadelphia: Temple Ursity Press, 1982.

Freund, Peter E. S., and Meredith B McGuire. *Health, Illness, and the Social*

Body: A Critical Sociology. 2nd ed. Englewood Cliffs: Prentice-Hall, 1995.

Gallagher, Nancy Elizabeth. *Egypt's Other Wars: Epidemics and the Politics of Public Health.* Syracuse: Syracuse University Press, 1990.

Geggus, David Patrick. *Slavery, War, and Revolution: The British Occupation of Saint Domingue, 1793–1798.* Oxford: Claredon Press, 1982.

Gentilini, Marc, and Jean-Pierre Nozais. "Expansion coloniale et santé." In *Histoire des médecins et pharmaciens de la Marine et des Colonies,* edited by Pierre Pluchon. Toulouse: Bibliothèque Historique Privat, 1985.

Gibbons v. Ogden, 22 U.S. 1 (1824).

Gobierno Civil de Santa Clara. *Memorias del estado de la Provincia y resumen de los trabajos realizados con observaciones e indicaciones sobre la marcha administrativa de la misma.* Havana: Imprenta "El Fígaro," 1900.

Gold Alvord, Thomas, Jr. "Is the Cuban Capable of Self-Government?" *Forum* 24 (1897–1898): 119–28.

Gómez, Máximo. *Cartas de Máximo Gómez.* Santo Domingo: Biblioteca Nacional, 1986.

———. *Diario de campaña del Mayor General Máximo Gómez, 1868–1899,* edited by Comisión del Archivo de Máximo Gómez. 2nd ed. Havana: Centro Superior Tecnológico Ceiba del Agua, 1942.

Gorgas, Marie D., and Burton J. Hendrick. *William Crawford Gorgas: His Life and Works.* New York: Doubleday, Page, and Co., 1924.

Gorgas, William C. *Sanitation in Panama.* New York: D. Appleton and Co., 1915.

Graf, Mercedes. "Women Physicians in the Spanish-American War." *Army History: The Professional Bulletin of Army History,* no. 56 (2002): 4–15, 28.

Gramsci, Antonio. *Selections from the Prison Notebooks.* Translated by Quintin Hoare and Geoffrey Nowell-Smith. New York: International Publishers, 1971.

Guicharnaud-Tolls, Michèle. *Regards sur Cuba au XIXe Siècle.* Paris: L'Harmattan, 1996.

Guiteras, Juan. "A False Alarm of Yellow Fever and How It Was Met by the Health Department." *Sanidad y beneficiencia* 6, no. 5 and 6 (1911): 664–67.

———. "Conferencia del Dr. Osler sobre 'La Nación y los Trópicos' y el Dr. Finlay." *Sanidad y beneficiencia* 3, no. 4 (1910): 313–17.

———. "El Dr. Carlos J. Finlay: Apuntes biográficos." *Anales de la Academia de Ciencias Médicas, Físicas y Naturales de La Habana* 48 (1911): 270–80.

———. "Health Conditions in Cuba," December 25, 1910, in "An Article from the 'Army and Navy Journal' and Reply of the Director of Public Health," *Sanidad y beneficiencia* 5, no. 1: 79–82.

———. "Informe sobre los candidatos Finlay y Agramonte al "Premio Nobel," Sección de Medicina." *Anales de la Academia de Ciencias Médicas, Físicas y Naturales de La Habana* 48 (March 1912): 605–12.

———. "La sanidad cubana y la opinión extranjera." *Sanidad y beneficiencia* 2, no. 1 (1909): 1–4.

———. "The Panama Canal and the Propagation of Epidemic Diseases." *Sanidad y beneficiencia* 6, no. 2 (1911): 220–21.

———. "The Supression of Yellow Fever in Cuba." *Medical Record* 75 (June 26, 1909): 1108–09.

———. "Tuberculosis in Cuba." *Sanidad y beneficiencia* 3, no. 1 and 2 (1910): 6–9.

Haller, John S. *American Medicine in Transition, 1840–1910.* Urbana: University of Illinois Press, 1981.

Harrison, Mark. *Public Health in British India: Anglo-Indian Preventive Medicine, 1859–1914.* Cambridge: Cambridge University Press, 1994.

Hazard, Samuel. *Cuba with Pen and Pencil.* London: Sampson Low, Son, and Marston, 1871.

Headrick, Daniel R. *The Tools of Empire: Technology and European Imperialism in the Nineteenth Century.* Oxford: Oxford University Press, 1981.

Healy, David F. *The United States in Cuba, 1898–1902: Generals, Politicians, and the Search for Policy.* Madison: University of Wisconsin Press, 1963.

———. *U.S. Expansionism: The Imperialist Urge in the 1890s.* Madison: University of Wisconsin Press, 1970.

Heiser, Victor. *An American Doctor's Odyssey: Adventures in Forty-five Countries.* New York: W. W. Norton and Co., 1936.

Hernández, José M. *Cuba and the United States: Intervention and Militarism, 1868–1933.* Austin: University of Texas Press, 1993.

Hill, G. Everett. "Colonel Waring on the Sanitation of Havana." *Forum* 26 (1899): 529–46.

Hill, Howard C. *Roosevelt and the Caribbean.* Chicago: University of Chicago Press, 1927.

Hill, Robert T. *Cuba and Porto Rico, with Other Islands of the West Indies.* New York: Century Co., 1909.

Hinton, Richard. "Cuban Reconstruction." *North American Review* 168, no. 56 (1899): 92–102.

Hitchman, James H. *Leonard Wood and Cuban Independence, 1898–1902.* The Hague: Martinus Nijhoff, 1971.

———. "The American Touch in Imperial Administration: Leonard Wood in Cuba, 1898–1902." *The Americas* 24, no. 4 (1968): 394–403.

———. "The Platt Amendment Revisited: A Bibliographical Survey." *The Americas* 23, no. 4 (1967): 343–69.

———. "Unfinished Business: Public Works in Cuba, 1898–1902." *The Americas* 31, no. 3 (1975): 335–59.

Hoganson, Kristin L. *Fighting for American Manhood: How Gender Politics Provoked the Spanish-American and Philippine-American Wars.* New Haven: Yale University Press, 1998.

"Homenaje al Dr. Carlos J. Finlay." *Sanidad y beneficiencia* 7, no. 6 (1912): 748–54.

Howard, Sidney, and Paul de Kruif. *Yellow Jack: A History.* New York: Harcourt, Brace, and Co., 1933.

Howe, Julia Ward. *A Trip to Cuba.* 2nd ed. (1st ed. 1890). New York: Negro Universities Press, 1969.

Hoy, Suellen. *Chasing Dirt: The American Pursuit of Cleanliness.* Oxford: Oxford University Press, 1995.

Huisman, Frank, and John Harley Warner, eds. *Locating Medical History: The Stories and Their Meanings.* Baltimore: Johns Hopkins University Press, 2004.

Humphreys, Margaret. "Hunting the Yellow Fever Germ: The Principle and Practice of Etiological Proof in Late Nineteenth-Century America." *Bulletin of the History of Medicine* 59 (1985): 361–82.

———. "Local Control Versus National Interest: The Debate over Southern Public Health, 1878–1884." *Journal of Southern History* 50, no. 3 (1984): 407–28.

———. "No Safe Place: Disease and Panic in American History." *American Literary History* 14, no. 4 (2002): 845–57.

———. *Yellow Fever and the South.* Baltimore: Johns Hopkins University Press, 1992.

Hunt, Nancy Rose. *A Colonial Lexicon of Birth Ritual, Medicalization, and Mobility in the Congo.* Durham: Duke University Press, 1999.

Ibarra, Jorge. *Cuba: 1898–1921, partidos políticos y clases sociales.* Havana: Editorial de Ciencias Sociales, 1992.

———. "Los mecanismos económicos del capital financiero obstaculizan la formación de la burguesía doméstica cubana (1898–1930)." *ISLAS* 79 (1984): 71.

———. *Máximo Gómez frente al imperio, 1898–1905.* Havana: Editorial de Ciencias Sociales, 2000.

———. *Prologue to Revolution: Cuba, 1898–1958.* Translated by Marjorie Moore. Boulder: Lynne Rienner Publishers, 1998.

Illich, Ivan. *Limits to Medicine.* London: Marion Boyars, 1976.

International Sanitary Bureau of the American Republics. *Transaction of the Third International Sanitary Conference of the American Republics.* Washington: International Bureau of the American Republics, 1907.

Jenkins, Jonathan S. "Life and Society in Old Cuba." *Century Magazine* 56–57, nos. 5–6, 1–2 (September–December 1898).

Jorgensen, Margareth. *Preliminary Inventory of the Records of the Military Government of Cuba (Record Group 140).* Washington: National Archives, 1962.

Joseph, Gilbert M., Catherine C. Legrand, and Ricardo D. Salvatore, eds. *Close Encounters of Empire: Writing the Cultural History of U.S.-Latin American Relations.* Durham: Duke University Press, 1998.

Keller, Allan. *The Spanish-American War: A Compact History.* New York: Hawthorn Books, 1969.

Keller, Kathryn J. "Racing Immunities: How Yellow Fever Gendered a Nation." Ph.D. diss., University of Washington, 2000.

Kelly, Howard A. *Walter Reed and Yellow Fever.* New York: McClure, Phillips and Co., 1906.

Kiple, Kenneth F. "Response to Sheldon Watts." *Journal of Social History* 34, no. 4 (2001): 968–74.

Kiple, Kenneth F., and Brian T. Higgins. "Yellow Fever and the Africanization of the Caribbean." In *Disease and Demography in the Americas,* edited by John W. Verano and Douglas H. Ubelaker. Washington: Smithsonian Institution Press, 1992.

Kramer, Paul A. *The Blood of Government: Race, Empire, the United States, and the Philippines.* Chapel Hill: University of North Carolina Press, 2006.

Le Prince, Joseph A., and A. J. Orenstein. *Mosquito Control in Panama: The Eradication of Malaria and Yellow Fever in Cuba and Panama.* New York: G. P. Putnam's Sons, Knickerbocker Press, 1916.

Le-Roy, Jorge. *Desenvolvimiento de la salud en Cuba durante los últimos cincuenta años (1871–1920).* Havana: Imprenta "La Moderna Poesía," 1922.

———. "Estadística sanitaria de Cuba: estudio de su población." *Cuba contemporánea* 7 (1915).

———. "La sanidad en Cuba: sus progresos." *Cuba contemporánea* 3 (1913).

———. "Public Health." In *Twentieth Century Impressions of Cuba,* edited by Reginal Lloyd. London, 1913.

———. "Reivindicación de la Gloria de Finlay." *Sanidad y beneficiencia* 32, no. 1, 2, and 3 (1927): 204–15.

Lee, Benjamin. "Do the Sanitary Interests of the United States Demand the Annexation of Cuba?" *Public Health Papers and Reports* 15 (1889): 47–52.

Lee, Fitzhugh. "Cuba under Spanish Rule." *McClure's Magazine,* June 1898, 99–114.

Lee, Fitzhugh, and Joseph Wheeler. *Cuba's Struggle against Spain.* New York: American Historical Press, 1899.

Lockmiller, David A. *Magoon in Cuba: A History of the Second Intervention, 1906–1909.* Chapel Hill: University of North Carolina Press, 1938.

López del Valle, José A. "Al Congreso de la Prensa Médica Latina." *Sanidad y beneficiencia* 32, nos. 1, 2, and 3 (1927): 202–03.

———. "Desenvolvimiento de la sanidad y la beneficiencia en Cuba durante los últimos diez y seis años (1899–1914)." In *Third Cuban National Medical Congress,* 1914.

———. "Discurso por el Dr. J. A. López del Valle, Secretario de la Junta Nacional de Sanidad y Beneficiencia y Profesor de Higiene de la Universidad Nacional, en el acto de desvelar las tarjas con los nombres de Finlay y de Guiteras." *Sanidad y beneficiencia* 32, nos. 1, 2, and 3 (1927): 163–82.

———. "La lucha contra el mosquito: Empleo de medios auxiliares, las biajacas, los guajacones." *Sanidad y beneficiencia* 3, no. 3 (1910): 224–36.

López Segrera, Francisco. *Cuba, cultura y sociedad (1510–1985).* Havana: Editorial Letras Cubanas, 1989.

———. *Cuba: Capitalismo dependiente y subdesarrollo (1510–1959).* Havana: Casa de las Américas, 1972.

———. *Sociología de la colonia y neocolonia cubana, 1510–1959.* Havana: Editorial de Ciencias Sociales, 1989.

Lorcin, Patricia M. E. "Imperialism, Colonial Identity, and Race in Algeria, 1830–1870: The Role of the French Medical Corps." *Isis* 90, no. 4 (1999): 653–79.

Löwy, Ilana. "What/who should be controlled? Opposition to yellow fever campaigns in Brazil, 1900–39." In *Western Medicine as Contested Knowl-*

edge, edited by Andrew Cunningham and Bridie Andrews. Manchester: Manchester University Press, 1997.

———. *Virus, moustiques et modernité: la fièvre jaune au Brésil, entre science et politique.* Paris: Éditions des archives contemporaines, 2001.

Lyons, Maryinez. "Sleeping Sickness, Colonial Medicine and Imperialism: Some Connections in the Belgian Congo." In *Disease, Medicine, and Empire: Perspectives on Western Medicine and the Experience of European Expansion,* edited by Roy MacLeod and Milton Lewis. New York: Routledge, 1988.

———. *The Colonial Disease: A Social History of Sleeping Sickness in Northern Zaire, 1900–1940.* Cambridge: Cambridge University Press, 1992.

Machado y Ortega, Luis. *La Enmienda Platt.* Havana: Imprenta "El Siglo XX," 1922.

Magoon, Charles E. *Republic of Cuba, Report of Provisional Administration from December 1st, 1907 to December 1st, 1908.* Havana: Rambla and Bouza, 1909.

———. *Republic of Cuba, Report of Provisional Administration from October 13th, 1906 to December 1st, 1907.* Havana: Rambla and Bouza, 1908.

Mannoni, Octave. *Prospero and Caliban: The Psychology of Colonization.* Translated by Pamela Powesland. New York: Frederick A. Praeger, 1956.

Márquez Sterling, Manuel. *Proceso histórico de la Enmienda Platt (1897–1934).* Havana: Imprenta "El Siglo XX," 1941.

Martínez, Oscar J., ed. *U.S.-Mexico Borderlands: Historical and Contemporary Perspectives.* Wilmington: Scholarly Resorces, 1996.

Martínez-Fortún Foyo, José A. "Historia de la medicina en Cuba (1840–1958)." *Cuadernos de la historia de la salud pública* 98, no. 1 (2005).

Matthews, Franklin. *The New-Born Cuba.* New York: Harper and Bros., 1899.

———. "The Reconstruction of Cuba," Parts 1–15. *Harper's Weekly* March–August, 1899.

McCarthy, Michael. "A Century of the US Army Yellow Fever Research." *Lancet* 357 (2001): 1772.

McGrew, Roderick E. *Russia and the Cholera, 1823–1832.* Madison: University of Wisconsin Press, 1965.

McNeill, John R. "Ecology, Epidemics, and Empires: Environmental Change and the Geopolitics of Tropical America, 1600–1825." *Environment and History* 5, no. 2 (1999): 175–84.

McNeill, William H. *Plagues and Peoples.* New York: Doubleday, 1976.

Memmi, Albert. *Portrait du colonisé.* Paris: Gallimard, 1985.

Mena, César A., and Fernando E. Cobelo. *Historia de la medicina en Cuba.* 2 vols. Miami: Ediciones Universal, 1992.

Ministerio de Ultramar. *Reglamento de Sanidad Marítima para la Isla de Cuba; Aprobado por Real orden de 8 de Marzo de 1893.* Madrid: Imprenta de La Viuda de M. Minuesa de los Ríos, 1893.

Mitchell, Timothy. *Rule of Experts: Egypt, Techno-Politics, Modernity.* Berkeley: University of California Press, 2002.

Moreno Fraginals, Manuel. *Cuba/España, España/Cuba: Historia común.* Barcelona: Crítica, 1995.

Morris, R. J. *Cholera 1832: The Social Response to an Epidemic*. New York: Holmes and Meier Publishers, 1976.

Naranjo Orovio, Consuelo, and Armando García González. *Medicina y racismo en Cuba: La ciencia ante la inmigración canaria en el siglo XX*. La Laguna, Tenerife: Centro de la Cultura Popular Canaria, 1996.

Needell, Jeffrey D. "The *Revolta Contra Vacina* of 1904: The Revolt against 'Modernization' in *Belle-Époque* Rio de Janeiro." *Hispanic American Historical Review* 67, no. 2 (1987): 233–69.

Neely v. Henkle, 180 U.S. 109 (1901).

Nelson, Wolfred. "Cuba in its Relation to the Southern United States; Its Danger as a Disease-Producing and Distributing Center." In *Tenth Biennial Report of the State Board of Health of California for the Fiscal Years from June 30, 1886, to June 30, 1888*. Sacramento: California State Board of Health, 1888.

Norman, Colin. "The Unsung Hero of Yellow Fever?" *Science* 223, no. 4643 (March 30, 1984): 1370–72.

Nuttall, George H. F. "On the Role of Insects, Arachnids and Myriapods as Carriers in the Spread of Bacteria and Parasitic Diseases of Man and Animals: A Critical and Historical Study." *Johns Hopkins Reports* 8 (1899–1900): 1–152.

Olmsted, Victor H., and Henry Gannett. *Cuba: Population, History and Resources*. Washington: United States Bureau of the Census, 1909.

Osgood, Robert Endicott. *Ideals and Self-Interest in America's Foreign Relations: The Great Transformation of the Twentieth Century*. Chicago: University of Chicago Press, 1953.

"Our Duty in Regard to Memphis." *Manufacturer and Builder* 2, no. 9 (1879): 204–05.

Palmer, Steven. *From Popular Medicine to Medical Populism: Doctors, Healers, and Public Power in Costa Rica, 1800–1940*. Durham: Duke University Press, 2003.

Parcero Torre, Celia María. *La pérdida de la Habana y las reformas borbónicas en Cuba, 1760–1773*. Valladolid: Junta de Castilla y León, Consejería de Educación y Cultura, 1998.

Patterson, Robert. "Dr. William Gorgas and His War with the Mosquito." *Canadian Medical Association Journal* 141 (1989): 596–99.

Paulsor. "La conquista científica de la fiebre amarilla." *Sanidad y beneficiencia* 5, no. 1 (1911): 106–08.

Pazos, José H. "Contribución al estudio de los mosquitos en Cuba." *Sanidad y beneficiencia* 2, no. 1 (1909): 28–51.

Peard, Julyan G. *Race, Place, and Medicine*. Durham: Duke University Press, 1999.

———. "Tropical Disorders and the Forging of the Brazilian Medical Identity, 1860–1890." *Hispanic American Historical Review* 77, no. 1 (1997): 1–44.

Pérez, Louis A., Jr. *Cuba and the United States: Ties of Singular Intimacy*. Athens: University of Georgia Press, 1990.

———. *Cuba between Empires, 1878–1902*. Pittsburgh: University of Pittsburgh Press, 1983.

————. *Cuba under the Platt Amendment, 1902–1934.* Pittsburgh: University of Pittsburgh Press, 1986.

————. *Cuba: Between Reform and Revolution.* 2nd ed. Oxford: Oxford University Press, 1995.

————. "Incurring a Debt of Gratitude: 1898 and the Moral Sources of United States Hegemony in Cuba." *American Historical Review* 104, no. 2 (1999): 356–98.

————. "Insurrection, Intervention, and the Transformation of Land Tenure Systems in Cuba, 1895–1902." *Hispanic American Historical Review* 65, no. 2 (1985): 229–54.

————. *On Becoming Cuban: Identity, Nationality, and Culture.* Chapel Hill: University of North Carolina Press, 1999.

————. *The War of 1898: The United States and Cuba in History and Historiography.* Chapel Hill: University of North Carolina Press, 1998.

Pierra, Fidel G. "The Present and Future of Cuba." *Forum* 22 (1897): 659–72.

Pirala, Antonio. *Anales de la Guerra de Cuba.* Madrid: Felipe González Rojas, 1895.

Poumier, María. "La vida cotidiana en las ciudades cubanas en 1898." *Universidad de La Habana* 196 (February–March 1972): 170–209.

Powell, John Harvey. *Bring Out Your Dead: The Great Plague of Yellow Fever in Philadelphia in 1793.* New York: Arno Press, 1949. Reprint, Philadelphia: University of Pennsylvania Press, 1993.

Powers, Ramon, and James N. Lieker. "Cholera Among the Plains Indians: Perceptions, Causes, Consequences." *Western Historical Quarterly* 29, no. 3 (1998): 317–40.

Prince, J. C. *Cuba Illustrated.* 6th ed. New York: Napoléon Thompson and Co., 1893–94.

Pruna Goodgall, Pedro M. *Ciencia y científicos en Cuba colonial, La Real Academia de Ciencias de La Habana.* Havana: Editorial Academia, 2001.

Quintana, Jorge. "Lo que costó a Cuba la Guerra de 1895." *Bohemia,* September 11, 1960, 4–6, 107–08.

Ramos Domínguez, Benito Narey, and Jorge Adereguía Henríquez. *Medicina social y salud pública en Cuba.* Havana: Editorial Pueblo y Educación, 1990.

Reaud, Ángel. "Epidemiología de la fiebre amarilla." *Salubridad y asistencia social* 51, no. 1–6 (1948): 3–31.

Reed, Walter. "The Propagation of Yellow Fever—Observations Based on Recent Researches." In *Yellow Fever: A Compilation of Various Publications,* edited by U.S. Senate. Washington: Government Printing Office, 1911 [1901].

Reed, Walter, James Carroll, and Arístides Agramonte. "The Etiology of Yellow Fever—An Additional Note." In *Yellow Fever: A Compilation of Various Publications,* edited by U.S. Senate. Washington: Government Printing Office, 1911 [1901].

Reed, Walter, James Carroll, Arístides Agramonte, and Jesse W. Lazear. "The Etiology of Yellow Fever—A Preliminary Note." In *Yellow Fever: A Compilation of Various Publications,* edited by U.S. Senate. Washington: Government Printing Office, 1911 [1900].

Reglamento de higiene para la ciudad de Puerto-Príncipe. Puerto-Príncipe: Tipografía "La Verdad," 1899.

Reid-Henry, Simon. *The Cuban Cure: Reason and Resistance in Global Science.* Chicago: University of Chicago Press, 2009.

Reiser, Stanley Joel. *Medicine and the Reign of Technology.* New York: Cambridge University Press, 1978.

República de Cuba. Senado. *Memoria de los trabajos realizados durante las cuatro legislaturas y sesión extraordinaria del primer período congresional, 1902–1904.* Havana: Imprenta y Papelería de Rambla, Bouza y Ca., 1918.

Robinson, Albert G. *Cuba Old and New.* 2nd ed. (1st ed., 1915). Connecticut: Negro Universities Press, 1970.

Rodríguez, José Ignacio. *Estudio histórico sobre el origen, desenvolvimiento y manifestaciones prácticas de la idea de la anexión de la Isla de Cuba a los Estados Unidos de América.* Havana: Imprenta La Propaganda Literaria, 1900.

Roig de Leuchsenring, Emilio. *Cuba no debe su independencia a los Estados Unidos.* Buenos Aires: Hemisferio, 1965.

———, ed. *Facetas de la vida de Cuba Republicana, 1902–1952,* Colección histórica cubana y americana. Havana: Oficina del Historiador de la Ciudad de La Habana, 1954.

———. *La lucha cubana por la república, contra la anexión y la Enmienda Platt, 1899–1902.* Havana: Oficina del Historiador de la Ciudad de La Habana, 1952.

———. *Médicos y medicina en Cuba.* Havana: Museo Histórico de las Ciencias Médicas "Carlos Finlay," 1965.

———. "Reiteradamente la obra de Finlay es negada o desconocida en los Estados Unidos," *Carteles* May 10, 1942, reprinted in Emilio Roig de Leuchsenring, *Médicos y medicina en Cuba.* Havana: Museo Histórico de las Ciencias Médicas "Carlos Finlay," 1965.

Rosenberg, Charles E. "Cholera in Nineteenth-Century Europe: A Tool for Social and Economic Analysis." *Comparative Studies in Society and History* 8, no. 4 (1966): 452–63.

Rosenberg, Charles E., and Janet Golden, eds. *Framing Disease: Studies in Cultural History.* New Brunswick: Rutgers University Press, 1992.

Rubens, Horatio Seymour. *Liberty: The Story of Cuba.* 2nd ed. Salem: Ayer Publishing, 1970.

Said, Edward W. *Orientalism.* New York: Pantheon Books, 1978.

"Sanitary Conditions in Cuba." *Medical Record* 75 (June 19, 1909): 1062.

Santos Fernández, Juan. "Contestación al discurso de recepción del Dr. Juan Guiteras en la Academia de Ciencias." *Anales de la Academia de Ciencias Médicas, Físicas y Naturales de La Habana* 48 (October 1911): 280–89.

Schoultz, Lars. *Beneath the United States: A History of U.S. Policy toward Latin America.* Cambridge: Harvard University Press, 1998.

Selections from Public Health Reports and Papers Presented at the Meetings of the American Public Health Association (1873–1883), edited by Barbara Gutmann Rosenkrantz, Public Health in America. New York: Arno Press, 1977.

Shaw, Albert. *International Bearings of American Policy.* Baltimore: Johns Hopkins University Press, 1943.

Slaughterhouse Cases, 83 U.S. 36 (1872).

Smallman-Raynor, Matthew, and Andrew D. Cliff. "Epidemic Diffusion Processes in a System of U.S. Military Camps: Transfer Diffusion and the Spread of Typhoid Fever in the Spanish-American War, 1898." *Annals of the Association of American Geographers* 91, no. 1 (2001): 71–91.

———. "The Spatial Dynamics of Epidemic Diseases in War and Peace: Cuba and the Insurrection against Spain, 1895–98." *Transactions of the Institute of British Geographers* 24, no. 3 (1999): 331–52.

Snowden, Frank M. "Cholera in Barletta 1910." *Past and Present* 132 (1991): 67–103.

———. *The Conquest of Malaria: Italy, 1900–1962.* New Haven: Yale University Press, 2006.

Sontag, Susan. *Illness as Metaphor.* New York: Farrar, Straus, and Giroux, 1977.

Souchon, Edmund. "True Origin of the Epidemic of Yellow Fever." *Journal of the American Medical Association* 35 (1900): 308–10.

Speer, James B., Jr. "Pestilence and Progress: Health Reform in Galveston and Houston during the Nineteenth Century." *Houston Review: History and Culture of the Gulf Coast* 2, no. 3 (1980): 120–32.

Spurr, David. *The Rhetoric of Empire: Colonial Discourse in Journalism, Travel Writing, and Imperial Administration.* Durham: Duke University Press, 1993.

Stepan, Nancy. "The Interplay between Socio-Economic Factors and Medical Science: Yellow Fever Research, Cuba and the United States." *Social Studies of Science* 8, no. 4 (1978): 397–423.

Sternberg, George. *Report on the Etiology and Prevention of Yellow Fever.* Washington: Government Printing Office, 1890.

Sutter, Paul S. "Nature's Agents or Agents of Empire? Entomological Workers and Environmental Change During the Construction of the Panama Canal." *Isis* 98, no. 4 (2007): 724–54.

"The Cost of Yellow Fever." *Journal of the American Medical Association* 29 (1897): 867.

"The Cuban Menace." *Medical Record* 75 (June 5, 1909): 975.

Thomas, Hugh. *Cuba: The Pursuit of Freedom.* New York: Harper and Row, Publishers, 1971.

Tone, John Lawrence. *War and Genocide in Cuba, 1895–1898.* Chapel Hill: University of North Carolina Press, 2006.

Trask, David F. *The War with Spain in 1898.* New York: Macmillan, 1981.

Treasury Department, Marine-Hospital Service. *Annual Report of the Surgeon-General of the Public Health and Marine-Hospital Service of the United States for the Fiscal Year 1903.* Washington: Government Printing Office, 1904.

———. *Annual Report of the Surgeon-General of the Public Health and Marine-Hospital Service of the United States for the Fiscal Year 1904.* Washington: Government Printing Office, 1904.

———. *Annual Report of the Surgeon-General of the Public Health and Marine-Hospital Service of the United States for the Fiscal Year 1905.* Washington: Government Printing Office, 1906.

———. *Annual Report of the Surgeon-General of the Public Health and Marine-Hospital Service of the United States for the Fiscal Year 1906.* Washington: Government Printing Office, 1907.

———. *Annual Report of the Surgeon-General of the Public Health and Marine-Hospital Service of the United States for the Fiscal Year 1907.* Washington: Government Printing Office, 1908.

———. *Annual Report of the Surgeon-General of the Public Health and Marine-Hospital Service of the United States for the Fiscal Year 1908.* Washington: Government Printing Office, 1909.

Truby, Albert E. *Memoir of Walter Reed: The Yellow Fever Episode.* New York: Paul B. Hoeber, 1943.

United States Adjutant General's Office. *Correspondence Relating to the War with Spain and Conditions Growing Out of the Same,* vol. 1. Washington: Government Printing Office, 1902.

United States Congress. House. *Annual Message of the President,* 56th Congress, 2nd Session, Document No. 1. Washington: Government Printing Office, 1901.

———. *Message of the President of the United States, Communicating to the two Houses of Congress, on the Relations of the United States to Spain by Reason of Warfare in the Island of Cuba,* 55th Congress, 2nd Session, Document No. 405. Washington: Government Printing Office, 1898.

United States Congress. Senate. *Proceedings of the Cuba and Florida Immigration Investigation, the Senate Committee on Immigration, the Senate Committee on Epidemic Diseases, and the House Committee on Immigration and Naturalization, Acting Jointly through Subcommittees at Havana, Cuba, and at Key West, Fla., December 28 to 31, 1892,* 52nd Congress, 2nd Session, Report No. 1263, Ser. 3072. Washington: Government Printing Office, 1893.

———. *Report of the Commission Appointed by the President to Investigate the Conduct of the War Department in the War with Spain.* 8 vols, 56th Congress, 1st Session, 8 vols., Ser. 3859–66. Washington: Government Printing Office, 1900.

———. *Supplemental Report of Provisional Governor of Cuba,* 61st Congress, 1st Session, No. 80, Ser. 5572. Washington: Government Printing Office, 1909.

———. *Transactions of the First General International Sanitary Convention of the American Republics, Held at the New Willard Hotel, Washington, D.C., December 2, 3, and 4, 1902, Under the Auspices of the Governing Board of the International Union of American Republics,* 57th Congress, 2nd Session, Document No. 169. Washington: Government Printing Office, 1901.

United States Department of State. *Papers Relating to the Foreign Relations of the United States, with the Annual Message of the President Transmitted to Congress, December 2, 1902.* Washington: Government Printing Office, 1903.

———. *Papers Relating to the Foreign Relations of the United States, with the Annual Message of the President Transmitted to Congress, December 5, 1898*. Washington: Government Printing Office, 1901.

———. *Papers Relating to the Foreign Relations of the United States, with the Annual Message of the President Transmitted to Congress, December 6, 1904*. Washington: Government Printing Office, 1905.

———. *Papers Relating to the Foreign Relations of the United States, with the Annual Message of the President Transmitted to Congress, December 1905*. Washington: Government Printing Office, 1906.

———. *Papers Relating to the Foreign Relations of the United States, with the Annual Message of the President Transmitted to Congress, December 1906*. Washington: Government Printing Office, 1909.

United States Marine-Hospital Service. *Annual Report of the Supervising Surgeon-General of the Marine-Hospital Service of the United States for the Fiscal Year 1895*. Washington: Government Printing Office, 1896.

———. *Annual Report of the Supervising Surgeon-General of the Marine-Hospital Service of the United States for the Fiscal Year 1896*. Washington: Government Printing Office, 1896.

———. *Annual Report of the Supervising Surgeon-General of the Marine-Hospital Service of the United States for the Fiscal Year 1897*. Washington: Government Printing Office, 1899.

———. *Annual Report of the Supervising Surgeon-General of the Marine-Hospital Service of the United States for the Fiscal Year 1898*. Washington: Government Printing Office, 1899.

———. *Annual Report of the Supervising Surgeon-General of the Marine-Hospital Service of the United States for the Fiscal Year 1899*. Washington: Government Printing Office, 1901.

———. *Report of the Commission of Medical Officers Detailed by Authority of the President to Investigate the Cause of Yellow Fever*. Washington: Government Printing Office, 1899.

United States Public Health and Marine-Hospital Service. *Annual Report of the Surgeon-General of the Public Health and Marine-Hospital Service of the United States for the Fiscal Year 1903*. Washington: Government Printing Office, 1904.

———. *Annual Report of the Surgeon-General of the Public Health and Marine-Hospital Service of the United States for the Fiscal Year 1904*. Washington: Government Printing Office, 1904.

———. *Annual Report of the Surgeon-General of the Public Health and Marine-Hospital Service of the United States for the Fiscal Year 1905*. Washington: Government Printing Office, 1906.

———. *Annual Report of the Surgeon-General of the Public Health and Marine-Hospital Service of the United States for the Fiscal Year 1906*. Washington: Government Printing Office, 1907.

———. *Annual Report of the Surgeon-General of the Public Health and Marine-Hospital Service of the United States for the Fiscal Year 1907*. Washington: Government Printing Office, 1908.

———. *Annual Report of the Surgeon-General of the Public Health and

Marine-Hospital Service of the United States for the Fiscal Year 1908.
Washington: Government Printing Office, 1909.

United States War Department. *Report of the Census of Cuba. 1899.* Washington: Government Printing Office, 1900.

Vinten-Johansen, Peter, Howard Brody, Nigel Paneth, Stephen Rachman, and Michael Rip. *Cholera, Chloroform, and the Science of Medicine: A Life of John Snow.* Oxford: Oxford University Press, 2003.

Warren, Andrew J. "Landmarks in the Conquest of Yellow Fever." In *Yellow Fever,* edited by George K. Strode, John C. Bugher, J. Austin Kerr, Hugh H. Smith, Kenneth C. Smithburn, Richard M. Taylor, Max Theiler, Andrew Warren and Loring Whitman. New York: McGraw-Hill Book Co., 1951.

Watts, Sheldon J. "Response to Kenneth Kiple." *Journal of Social History* 34, no. 4 (2001): 975–76.

———. "Yellow Fever Immunities in West Africa and the Americas in the Age of Slavery and Beyond: A Reappraisal." *Journal of Social History* 34, no. 4 (2001): 955.

Welch, Jr., Robert E. "William McKinley: Reluctant Warrior, Cautious Imperialist." In *Traditions and Values: American Diplomacy, 1865–1945,* edited by Norman A. Graebner. Lanham, MD: University Press of America, 1985.

Welsh, Osgood. "Cuba as Seen from the Inside." *Century Magazine* 54, no. 4 (August 1898): 586–93.

Williams, Beryl, and Samuel Epstein. *William Crawford Gorgas: Tropic Fever Fighter.* New York: Julian Massner, 1953.

Williams, Patrick, and Laura Chrisman, eds. *Colonial Discourse and Postcolonial Theory: A Reader.* New York: Harvest Wheatsheaf, 1994.

Williams, Ralph Chester. *The United States Public Health Service, 1798–1950.* Washington: Commissioned Officers Association of the United States Public Health Service, 1951.

Wisan, Joseph E. *The Cuban Crisis as Reflected in the New York Press (1895–1898).* New York: Columbia University Press, 1934.

Wood, Leonard. *Civil Report of Brigadier General Leonard Wood, Military Governor of Cuba (1902).* Washington: Government Printing Office, 1902.

———. *Civil Report of Major General Leonard Wood, Military Governor of Cuba, (1900) for the Period from December 20th, 1899 to December 31st 1900.* 12 vols. Washington: Government Printing Office, 1901.

Woodworth, J. M. "A Brief Review of the Organization and Purpose of the Yellow Fever Commission." *Public Health Reports and Papers Presented at the Meetings of the American Public Health Association* 4 (1877–78).

Worboys, Michael. "Manson, Ross and Colonial Medical Policy: Tropical Medicine in London and Liverpool, 1899–1914." In *Disease, Medicine, and Empire: Perspectives on Western Medicine and the Experience of European Expansion,* edited by Roy MacLeod and Milton Lewis. New York: Routledge, 1988.

Wyman, Walter. "Some Lessons of the Yellow Fever Epidemic." *Forum* 24, no. 3 (1897): 282–89.

Zulawski, Ann. *Unequal Cures: Public Health and Political Change in Bolivia, 1900–1950.* Durham: Duke University Press, 2007.

Index